Practical Law of Attraction

The Science of Attracting More of What You Want
(Health, Wealth, and Love)

Nick Whitley

Copyright © 2020 - All Rights Reserved.

The content contained within this book may not be reproduced, duplicated or transmitted without direct written permission from the author or the publisher.

Under no circumstances will any blame or legal responsibility be held against the publisher, or author, for any damages, reparation, or monetary loss due to the information contained within this book. Either directly or indirectly.

Legal Notice:

This book is copyright protected. This book is only for personal use. You cannot amend, distribute, sell, use, quote or paraphrase any part, or the content within this book, without the consent of the author or publisher.

Disclaimer Notice:

Please note the information contained within this document is for educational and entertainment purposes only. All effort has been executed to present accurate, up to date, and reliable, complete information. No warranties of any kind are declared or implied. Readers acknowledge that the author is not engaging in the rendering of legal, financial, medical or professional advice. The content within this book has been derived from various sources. Please consult a licensed professional before attempting any techniques outlined in this book.

By reading this document, the reader agrees that under no circumstances is the author responsible for any losses, direct or indirect, which are incurred as a result of the use of information contained within this document, including, but not limited to, — errors, omissions, or inaccuracies.

Table of Contents

Prologue 5

PARABLE: THE ADVENTURER AND THE ANSWER 6

Introduction: The Ice Cream Principle & Getting Everything You Want 7

Chapter 1: Your Mission - The ONE Thing You Need to Do Before Anything Else 17

Chapter 2: Law of Attraction - The Foundation of Everything You Bring into Your Life 21

Chapter 3: The Truth About the Law of Attraction That Nobody Ever Told You 29

Chapter 4: The Real Reason It Hasn't Worked for You Yet 37

Chapter 5: Paving Your Way to Success 45

Chapter 6: Deciding What You Want (For Real, This Time) 53

Chapter 7: Creating the State of Being for Manifesting Your Desires 59

Chapter 8: What to Expect Before You Begin (3 Key Traps to Watch Out For) 63

Chapter 9: Signaling the Universe Through Gratitude 69

Chapter 10: The Stacking Method 73

Chapter 11: The Time-Lapse Method 77

Chapter 12: Gratitude Attraction Boosters 81

Chapter 13: The Blitz Method 85

Chapter 14: The Discount Trigger Method... 89

Chapter 15: Why These Methods Work.. 93

Chapter 16: The Pennies to Millions Method 101

Chapter 17: The Unstoppable Power of Scripting............................. 105

Chapter 18: The Story Scripting Method.. 111

Chapter 19: The Statement Scripting Method..................................... 119

Chapter 20: The "Why It's So Great" Scripting Method................. 123

Chapter 21: Guidelines and Tips for High-Impact Scripting........ 127

Chapter 22: The Power (And Simplicity) of Visualization............ 135

Chapter 23: The Manifestation Method Menu 139

Chapter 24: An Easy Way to Meditate... 155

Chapter 25: The Ultimate Money Meditation Method................... 157

Chapter 26: The Walking Meditation Method.................................... 161

Chapter 27: Strategies for Sticking with It 165

Chapter 28: Finding A "Why" That Makes Everything Work...... 179

Chapter 29: Making Yourself Worthy (And Making Sure the Universe Knows It) 185

Chapter 30: You've Been Chosen... 195

Epilogue: Gravity of the Cosmos 203

A QUICK NOTE FROM ANDREW:.. 213

Prologue

Dear Reader, thank you for picking up Practical Law of Attraction! I know you could have chosen anything else in the world, but something clicked inside you when you saw the cover, and a little voice inside whispered "that one!"

You'll understand why you found this book shortly. But I want to quickly show my gratitude by giving you a fun extra bonus right now.

You see, not long after putting the finishing touches on this book, inspiration struck, and I ended up writing a little more than I was expecting. And now I've got this bonus chapter to share that doesn't really fit in with the flow of everything else in the book. But it's a super helpful lesson, and it'll really complement everything that you're about to learn in the pages to follow.

It's titled: "Knowing When To Hand Over Control And Let The Universe Do The Work For You"

To read it at any time, simply head over to:

www.LastLOABook.com

And download it at your convenience.

It's certainly not required reading, but it's one of my favorite Law of Attraction explanations. And it'll really help you understand more of why the methods in this book will be so useful to you. So you definitely won't want to miss it.

Thanks, and enjoy!

P.S. I included a few other goodies with the bonus chapter as well, and I'll tell you all about them at the very end of this book. But we'll get there soon enough. In the meantime, please enjoy Practical Law of Attraction! Life is about to get awesome.

PARABLE: THE ADVENTURER AND THE ANSWER

There was once a kind and curious adventurer who stumbled upon a mysterious book about the nature of the Universe. They opened to the first page and read the words:

Thoughts become reality. Like attracts like.

The thoughts that you think (and the emotions that you feel about those thoughts) energetically magnetize and attract the people, things, circumstances, and outcomes that you experience.

What you think about in your mind becomes your physical reality.

Intrigued, this adventurer turned the page and kept reading. They learned all about the Law of Attraction, but not in the way they were expecting. This was new. This went in a completely different direction than they thought it would after reading those first few words.

They discovered the last missing pieces of a puzzle they didn't even realize they were trying to solve. And everything finally changed for them.

The adventurer in this story is you.

So turn the page.

Introduction: The Ice Cream Principle & Getting Everything You Want

What if everything you've ever wanted really was just a thought away?

What if you could easily manifest the money, relationships, health, success, and life you always desired?

And what if there really was a universal principle known as "The Law of Attraction" that made it all possible?

If all of this really was true, and every wish you've ever made really was within your grasp... Then why are you still waiting for everything to come? And how do you finally get it?

This book was written to answer those questions.

It was written because -- while you may not realize this yet -- you actually already have everything you need to unlock your dreams and manifest your desires.

And yet you still haven't managed to do it.

So it's time for a new level of clarity to help you finally achieve the results you were promised a long time ago -- so that you'll never have to read another "Law of Attraction" book again.

No More Research. No More Questions.No More Waiting.

This is it. Everything you need to create the change you've been seeking and attract everything you want in life. You're finally going to do this (no, really - you ARE!).

And it's all going to happen in a way that just wasn't possible with your previous understanding of how the Universe works.

Those other books weren't wrong, by the way. In fact, a lot of them were brilliant. But there was either a missing piece in their explanation or a simple glitch in your understanding (or maybe a combination of both) that resulted in you not properly doing what they taught you to.

For whatever reason, you just couldn't find a way to get the lessons that they shared to work for you. But whatever that reason might be, it's no longer something you need to worry about. This is Practical Law of Attraction.

And no matter how much or how little you already know about this universal principle, it's time to finally use it the way it was always meant to be used.

Two Types - Which One Are You?

There are two types of people who find their way to this book:

Those who are brand new to the Law of Attraction ...and those who've been aware of it for a long time, but just haven't found a way to put all the pieces together.

Regardless of which category you fall into, you're going to be just fine. If this is your first Law of Attraction book, you've got yourself the perfect jumping on point. Most readers don't find this material until after they've already gone through countless other books and programs trying to somehow make this all "work" for them.

But starting with what's in this book will save you years of your life, as well as hundreds (if not thousands) of dollars -- to say nothing of the frustration, uncertainty, overwhelm, and doubt that more experienced readers have unfortunately already had to endure.

You're going to leapfrog past all of that.

And it's not that those other books weren't absolutely fantastic in their own way. Or that they didn't teach accurate information. It's just that there's usually one or two critical missing pieces that they inadvertently seem to leave out, which we'll talk about soon.

If this isn't your first Law of Attraction book, you understand what I mean. You know what it's like to be blown away by these ideas, learn amazing techniques, try them out, BEGIN to make progress, and then somehow always end up hitting a wall before you get too far.

The good news is you're finally about to get those last remaining pieces of the puzzle to make this work. And you're going to understand why it hasn't happened for you until now. Not only will this replace all the other Law of Attraction books, but it'll also replace all the love programs, money programs, meditation courses -- everything.

You'll no longer need them because everything is already here for you in these pages.

And if you find yourself even slightly tempted to buy more Law of Attraction books after this one, that may be a crucial sign to you that you're procrastinating because you have doubts that the Law actually works ...and you don't want to face the hopelessness of that kind of reality. Or maybe you know it's real, but you doubt your own worthiness on some level, and you're worried that the Universe isn't listening to you.

In other words, there may be a block there, and through the presentation of this book's content, we'll be addressing it for you (and solving it as well).

The reasons you haven't yet attracted the life you want might seem impossible to figure out right now, but they're way simpler than you think.

And once you understand what they are, you'll never be able to go back. This leaves us with two important questions:

What are these reasons and what can we do about them?

Why The Law of Attraction Hasn't Given You The Life of Your Dreams ...Yet!

Every Law of Attraction book you've EVER read was right.

You have more power than you realize. The Universe really IS in your corner. And the techniques that are already out there for attracting what you want ...are actually correct.

So why haven't any of them worked?

Why don't you have what you want?

This is part of what we'll cover (and overcome) in this book, but the long and short of it is that there are circumstances (that you're not entirely aware of) which are preventing you from using the techniques with the enthusiasm AND consistency that are needed. For example, one of your biggest hurdles right now is you still don't believe in the Law of Attraction 100%. Even if you think you do.

It's human nature. If you can't actually "see" the Law of Attraction happening, there's always going to be a subtle level of doubt holding you back until you actually get enough evidence of it working for you. You might even believe that it works for certain people in certain situations ...but you still don't believe it works reliably for YOU.

After all, if you really had no doubts and truly wanted things in your life to improve, NOTHING would stop you from sticking with it every single day until it happened.

But instead, most people seem perfectly fine reading all the books and doing all the programs ...until it's actually time to use what they learn.

That's when they hesitate. They take "some" action, but not nearly enough. Then they get frustrated, they look for "a better book" ...and the cycle repeats all over again. Meanwhile, that nagging question of "what if it doesn't really work?" always seems to be there on some level.

And unfortunately, living with that uncertainty is a way better option to them than taking a leap of faith, going all in with the methods they've learned ...but then losing all hope if it turns out that the Law of Attraction wasn't real after all. Even worse than that is the worry that they're simply not good enough, and that their "unworthiness" is the reason it's not working for them.

This is why the techniques you use will need to be able to bypass these fears and doubts -- at least until you experience enough evidence to know at your very core that this really works.

If this doesn't make complete sense yet, think of it as if you were trying to get in shape...

The Workout You Can Never Seem To Do

Have you ever asked yourself why most people don't work out every day? Or why some can barely bring themselves to do it even once a year?

After all, when you think about it, daily exercise is one of the healthiest activities out there. But if you ask most people why they can't manage to follow even an occasional exercise routine, they've always got an answer like:

- They tried it for a little while, but didn't get results quickly enough, so they stopped.

- They don't have enough time to do it.
- It's just not fun for them, so they're really not motivated to stick with it.
- They aren't sure if they're doing it right, and they lack confidence.
- The exercises seem too complicated.
- The exercises seem too simple, so they probably don't even work -- so why bother?
- They don't believe working out can really help them as much as it's helped other people.
- They want to work out, but for some reason, they never seem to be able to just start.

...Or maybe they don't even know the reason. All they know is they fail every time they try. And this is exactly what happens to people who read Law of Attraction books and try to do 'manifesting' exercises every day.

Unless this is your first Law of Attraction book (and again, if it is, you're about to save A LOT of time and money), at least half of that list is probably very familiar to you.

And the sad thing is that you've had access to perfectly good techniques for attracting what you want in your life this entire time.

But it's like that workout that you know you should do, but you constantly put off anyway. You simply haven't found an exercise that you actually enjoy enough to do every day.

And just like with working out, when it comes to Law of Attraction techniques, you can't just do them every so often and expect to get results. They have to be a daily part of your life.

And knowing they "have to" do it every day is what frustrates people the most and makes them give up before they even start.

And let's be honest with ourselves here -- after all the books, all the programs, and all the opportunities you've already had to finally get a handle on this -- you're not going to do ANY techniques on a daily basis UNLESS you actually enjoy them, UNLESS you know how to do them well, UNLESS you believe in them, and UNLESS you can actually appreciate the journey you'll be on while you're attracting your desires and manifesting your dreams.

THIS IS THE KEY to what you'll be getting in the pages to follow. Because if there's ONE piece all those other books have apparently missed so far -- it's providing a presentation and explanation that will help you enjoy, understand, and experience TRUE patience with these Law of Attraction methods -- so that you'll finally actually use them without it feeling like a constant chore!

The PERFECT Ice Cream

Let's go back to the example of working out.

There are lots of reasons why doing it every day is a good idea.

But let's just say for the purposes of our example that the goal of working out is to lose weight, get in shape, and have a fit healthy body. We know that 'working out' is a proven solution for doing all of this -- which is bad news for a lot of people, because working out isn't really that fun for them.

But what if "working out" wasn't the ONLY way to get in shape?

What if someone could wave a magic wand and invent a special type of magic ice cream -- that had ALL the positive qualities that regular ice cream has, NONE of the negative qualities, and also somehow had the EXACT same effect on your body as working out did -- even with just one spoonful a day? (If you're not a fan of ice cream -- think pizza, pancakes, cookies, etc.)

Think about all the advantages this would give you, and why it would be so easy to 'do':

- You enjoy it.
- You have no trouble doing it.
- It doesn't feel like an intrusion on your day.
- You never get tired of it.
- You never get bored with it.
- ...and best of all, you even look forward to it!

THAT'S what the manifestation methods in this book have been designed to be for you. The whole point of them is that they're actually their own reward. Yes, they're a means to an end -- a way to get what you want.

But they're also never a chore, and even if they weren't helping you attract what you want, you'd still enjoy doing them. So you know you can confidently stick with them until whatever you want manifests, no matter how slowly or quickly your results come.

This is why they're the perfect solution. You need a set of tools that you know you can use every single day (without it feeling like an obligation) because THAT is what's required for the Law of Attraction to work.

This is why the Law of Attraction hasn't seemed to work for a lot of people yet. They just haven't had access to the right combination of information, strategy, and methods.

But now you do.

You're Holding Everything You Need

In Your Hands Right Now.

Unless this really is your first Law of Attraction book, you should expect some of what you read here to already be familiar, some to be completely new, and some to give original perspectives on things you already thought you knew. Ultimately, though, the real value here will be the level of clarity and purpose you achieve as you finally clear out any remaining fear and doubt that was holding you back this whole time.

This book was written with the expectation that every reader should have their hand held as much as they personally need for them to actually be able to use these methods in a confident, comfortable, and consistent way.

Again, the methods have to be fun. Like eating ice cream.

And they will be.

Everything's Going To Make Sense

...And Everything's Going To Be Okay.

Remember, the value here is not only in the knowledge being presented, but in the methods that will help you use that knowledge. You'll need both, so have patience as you read through everything.

Later chapters will teach you some of the world's premiere-level techniques for manifesting your desires and attracting a life that you love. And you'll have plenty to choose from in case you need variety.

But you'll want to take your time getting there and make sure you read everything leading up to them first. Everything here is in a very specific order for a reason. And while I didn't waste pages on pointless filler, I was as thorough as I could be to make sure you have everything you need.

In fact, the only in-depth Law of Attraction resource I offer besides this book is an interactive advanced level program for those who want daily guidance and faster momentum without having to figure everything out by themselves (at the end of the book, I'll give you a link to get the first couple days for free so you can get your own boost of momentum, along with a few other surprises that you'll absolutely love).

I occasionally do one-on-one phone consultations for those who need the personal attention, and one or two other things devoted to a specific topic, but when it comes to the Law of Attraction as a full and complete category -- this book is the big one.

In other words, everything's here for you between these pages. I held nothing back. All you need to do is read it and follow the easy instructions. Everything else will literally take care of itself for you.

Let's dive in so you can find out for yourself.

Chapter 1: Your Mission - The ONE Thing You Need to Do Before Anything Else

There's a reason you haven't been able to make the Law of Attraction work for you yet. And now that you've read this book's introduction, it's probably becoming more obvious to you.

But just in case it's not clear enough yet, let's not mince words -- You're sabotaging yourself without realizing it.

Lucky for you, this doesn't have to keep happening. You can easily break the unconscious patterns that have been holding you back. After all, the Law of Attraction WORKS. And the Universe WANTS you to have what you desire! In fact, everything you want... literally wants you right back! And all you need to do in order to get it ...is simply get out of your own way.

THAT'S your mission. And once you accomplish it, everything else resolves itself pretty quickly. You see, the Law of Attraction is designed to make things predictable and simple for you. And if you could just flip a switch right now and make choices that are in harmony with how it already works, everything would suddenly get a LOT easier. Fortunately, flipping this switch is not only possible -- it's exactly what the manifestation methods in this book are here to help you do.

Unfortunately, since a lot of our past experiences have taught us to view the world with a mindset of scarcity, we usually don't really think this is possible and we aren't sure where to begin.

Instead, we hold ourselves back with limiting beliefs that are so second-nature by now that they're mostly invisible. You don't even notice them keeping you down.

This is where self-sabotage comes in, and it brings us back to the two main challenges we've got in front of us as we approach this mission of getting out of our own way:

1 - Using the easy techniques in this book with clarity, confidence, and enthusiasm.

2 - Doing them consistently enough for the things that we want to begin manifesting.

This would all be way simpler if you weren't already conditioned from childhood to view everything around you through the lens of scarcity, struggle, and limitation. In fact, if only you could wave a magic wand and instantly forget every doubt that you ever had about yourself, everything in your life would literally change overnight.

But since you're most likely not simply going to dissolve your limiting beliefs overnight, you need manifestation methods that you can enjoy enough to do consistently anyway.

You also need a few additional insights about how and why your mind works the way it does so that you can catch yourself whenever a roadblock is thrown in front of you.

For example, if you've read through any other Law of Attraction book, you've probably already been told things like:

- "Fully believe it is yours, and it will be."

- "Change the inside first, and the outside will change as a result."

- "All you have to do is be aligned with what you want, and you can have it."

But here's the problem that nobody really talks about: Telling you to do something (in order to get a specific desired result) ISN'T exactly useful ...if you don't know HOW to do the thing that you're being told to do.

For instance, telling you that you need to be "aligned" with your goals in order to attract and receive them isn't really helpful advice. Sure, the word "aligned" is simple and easy to understand intellectually. But it can also be an extremely frustrating topic because Law of Attraction books will tell you "you just have to be aligned" ...and then say nothing else about it. But what EXACTLY does "aligned" even mean???

That's like saying "hey, do you want to touch the sun? No problem - just jump really, really high." You're still left wondering HOW to jump that high. There's no clarity on how to actually accomplish this. This is one of the biggest reasons people have so much trouble using the Law of Attraction and end up buying more books trying to figure everything out.

But this is also where the book you're holding in your hands is finally different. You see, anytime you're told to be "aligned" or "just believe" or "change the inside first" ...you actually don't have to manually do anything! The manifestation methods in this book will do it FOR you.

The ONLY thing you need to do ...is get out of your own way by being open-minded enough to give these techniques an honest try. THAT'S THE WHOLE TRICK. And miracles will soon follow. Don't fall into the trap of thinking you've already tried something from this book before.

Until you've tried the techniques using the instructions you read here, you haven't given them a real chance. Also, don't fall into the trap of thinking you're not worthy of everything you want. You ARE worthy, and this is one of the biggest issues that people block themselves with. We'll make sure to address this in one of the final chapters and show you how to get past it once and for all.

Finally, don't fall into the trap of ever thinking this is hopeless or it can't be done. There's a way to do it, and the way has been provided. You only have to do your part, and the rest will be done for you. Think about what you're doing here like building muscle. You can't just grit your teeth, focus really hard, and "will" your muscles to grow. But you CAN lift weights to TRIGGER their growth.

In that same way, the manifestation methods in this book will TRIGGER the energetic attraction of what you want. They'll trigger the alignment for you. They'll trigger the manifestation. They'll trigger the result. Only unlike lifting weights, these methods won't be annoying, tiring, inconvenient, or painful.

You've had access to an unparalleled level of abundance this whole time. You just haven't known how to get to it yet. So just stay out of your own way, and keep reading. The way will be shown to you.

Chapter 2: Law of Attraction - The Foundation of Everything You Bring into Your Life

Are you ready to learn the blueprint for having everything you want in life? It all begins with one simple LAW.

And while you most likely knew what the Law of Attraction was before you found this book, let's have one final refresher to make sure we understand everything in the same way.

LAW OF ATTRACTION: THE SHORT VERSION

You attract whatever you give your energy, attention, and focus to. If you're thinking about it, you're magnetizing it to your life -- whether it's positive or negative.

Your focus may be on something you want. Or it may be on something you don't want (or the lack of what you want).

This is simply the way the Universe works. And once you accept it and live your life based on this truth, things you never previously dreamt of suddenly become possible.

LAW OF ATTRACTION: THE SLIGHTLY LONGER VERSION

Everything is energy.

I'll say that one more time because people often understand this intellectually when they hear it, but then rarely stop to consider what the implications of it really are.

So, again...

Everything is energy.

EVERYTHING.

Including your thoughts.

YOU are made up entirely of energy. The chair you're sitting in is made up of the SAME kind of energy. The planets and stars and everything else in existence is also made up of the same kind of energy.

And everything that's made of energy vibrates at a certain unique "frequency."

EVERYTHING

Including your thoughts.

The only difference between a person and a peanut is in how the energy of each one is "organized" into physical reality (i.e. the rate of their vibrational frequency). But the core foundation is all the same. And if you look at anything 'physical' under a microscope, you'll see that it isn't solid in the way you've always been led to believe.

Instead, it's all vibrating at its own specific frequency. And the 'rate' or 'vibration' of that frequency determines how 'solid' it SEEMS from the perspective of your body's physical senses. This means that the reality around you is really just a result of how your physical senses interpret the vibrations of whatever you encounter.

This is how a rock and a flower can be made up of the same energy and yet still be experienced very differently in the manifested physical plane that you're living in. It's also how emotions, outcomes, events, circumstances, and anything else that seems "intangible" (according to how you view reality) can all also each be made up of the same foundational energy. Here's where it gets interesting...

Since everything is energy ...and everything is connected at that foundational energetic level ...you are technically connected to the ENTIRE universe around you. And the entire Universe (including the energy of everything that you want!!) is connected back to you. Because of this connection to everything within it, the Universe knows EVERYTHING.

It "knows" everything you're thinking.

It "knows" the solution to every problem you have.

It "knows" the fastest, easiest, most enjoyable way for you to experience those solutions.

AND it has the means to magnetize similar vibrational patterns in order to put you and those solutions together in your physical reality. All it needs from you is to be "aligned" with those solutions (and remember - the techniques in this book will handle that alignment for you).

But here's the key to all of this:

The Universe is ALWAYS listening - even if you aren't.

It's listening to what you think.

It's listening to what you say.

It's listening to what you do.

So if you say you're waiting for the love of your life to find you, but you haven't cleared out space in your closet for them, the Universe sees the contradiction. If people ask you how you're doing and your answer is "I'm hanging in there" -- the Universe hears you "saying" that your life is boring, mediocre, and probably a bit of a struggle.

And -- here's a big one -- if you keep buying more and more Law of Attraction books -- UNLESS you're buying them because you genuinely enjoy their positivity and you simply like reading about it -- the Universe knows that you didn't have enough faith in the last book ...or enough faith in yourself ...OR enough faith in the Law of Attraction ...to finally use it and manifest your biggest dreams. (If any of this is true, don't worry -- it's going to be okay. With what you're reading now, you're finally on the cusp of everything you've ever wanted. It all begins with the awareness you're being given right now.)

So if the Universe is ALWAYS listening, that means you're ALWAYS using the Law of Attraction.

You're using it whether you realize it or not.

You're using it whether you want to or not.

And you're using it whether you like what you're attracting into your life or not.

Not being aware of the Law of Attraction doesn't keep it from happening. Like it or not, we're attracting and creating our reality every single moment of every single day. You've been creating your own reality on autopilot this entire time -- since the day you were born.

And now that you realize this, you have a golden opportunity to use your thoughts, words, and emotions to consciously take control and create the life you've always wanted (if that feels daunting, remember -- the methods in this book will do this for you as long as you actually use them!).

You're A Magnet.

We're all "magnets." And what we focus on is magnetized to us. We think thoughts, and those thoughts vibrate (remember, everything is energy -- and energy vibrates). Through that vibration, since like attracts like, those thoughts then draw in other energy with more and more momentum until the "thing" that was being magnetized finally "pops" into our manifested physical reality.

Our energetic vibrations give off signals which attract other 'like' signals back to us. And whether it's on purpose or not, we always end up aligning to the frequency of whatever reality we've been "thinking" about. We then get that outcome manifested into our physical world. This is 'law' -- and it's as reliable as gravity.

These manifestations take time, of course. That's just the way it is. Rome wasn't built in a day, that car you're driving wasn't created overnight, and the money you've been wanting for years probably won't instantly pop into your bank account after thinking about it for only 5 seconds.

For those things that seem to take longer than they should, there's usually a push-pull of energy going on in the background because some of your thoughts are contradicting others on a subconscious level without you even realizing it.

Ultimately, though, either "what you want" is going to have the edge of momentum and manifest into your physical reality ...or the "lack of what you want" is going to materialize instead. It all comes down to tipping the scales one way or another, and again, that's exactly what the manifestation methods in this book were designed for (including how to habitually do them WITHOUT it feeling like a chore or some inconvenient obligation). But first, it's important for you to understand that the Universe doesn't care what choice you make -- it only follows the instructions that you give it.

The Disinterested Donut Guy

Imagine you're in a donut shop placing an order that includes a Sugar Coated, a Glazed, a Jelly-Filled, a Chocolate Frosted, and a few others. The clerk behind the counter isn't wondering whether you'll actually enjoy any of these donuts. All he's hearing is your order.

He doesn't know if you're allergic to jelly. He doesn't care if you dislike chocolate. All he knows is that you "asked" for them. He's completely disinterested in whether you like what you get.

This is how it works with the Universe. Thinking about something (or the lack of something) is your energetic way of "asking" for it to become an outcome in your reality. So if you're reading this and saying "this makes no sense, I think about money ALL the time! Where's muh money!?" -- you might want to carefully consider whether you were REALLY thinking about money ...or if you were instead thinking about the LACK of money. This is where your emotions come in and really help you sort this all out.

Good/Positive Emotions = Desired Outcomes Are On The Way

Bad/Negative Emotions = Unwanted Outcomes Are On The Way

How you feel when you're thinking about anything is your clear indication of whether something you want is on the way to your reality ...or whether something you DON'T want will be there instead. In fact, it's impossible for you to align with certain thoughts and feelings without also creating their corresponding outcomes in your physical reality.

So as long as you choose the right thoughts in a way that will give you the right feelings, your happiness and success become inevitable.

In other words, there's a difference between thinking of money and feeling hopeful, happy, confident, reassured, comfortable, at ease, and generally positive (which means your money is on the way)...

...and thinking of money and feeling concern, worry, stress, frustration, sadness, impatience, disappointment, or any other negative emotions (which means you're keeping the money from coming to you).

This obviously goes for everything else in your life, including relationships, business, health, and every other topic in between. The really good news is that if you've been focused negatively on what you don't want for a very long time, it's much easier to turn the momentum around in your favor than you might think.

The Power and Leverage of Positivity

Positive thoughts and emotions have much more power than negative ones. This is why it's so easy to really pick up steam toward the life you want in spite of any negative thoughts or emotions you've been experiencing until now. Having a pure positive focus even once a day for only 60 seconds can (and does) make a significant difference in what you attract. So with the right techniques, we can easily begin to rewire our neural pathways for thinking in a much healthier way on autopilot.

Those healthier thoughts will then make us feel more positive emotions, and those emotions will add fuel to the manifestation process...until our desired result and outcome finally arrives in our physical reality. A huge key in all of this is understanding how far your energetic reach really is.

If you're really going to be successful, you need to understand whether you can only influence a little around you or whether you can influence a lot. The truth may surprise you. And we'll address this and more in the next chapter.

Chapter 3: The Truth About the Law of Attraction That Nobody Ever Told You

Take a quick moment right now, close your eyes, and for the next ten seconds take a few deep easy breaths picturing yourself on a beach holding hands with someone you're deeply in love with.

...that moment you just experienced (along with the thoughts behind it) literally just shot out and instantly touched the furthest reaches of the Universe. This is no exaggeration.

It's a bit like when you're on a phone call with someone on a completely different continent. Your phone transmits the signal of your voice through satellite towers and the person on the other end hears what you say to them INSTANTLY.

That's how fast the visualization of you on the beach from a minute ago transmitted across the galaxy. Think of the enormity of this! You may not consciously notice it happening ...but it IS happening.

It's like a dog whistle. You never hear any sound coming out of it, but every canine around you reacts anyway. So it must be there. It's just on a frequency of vibration that your senses aren't designed to detect or interpret in your reality. This is SO important, and if you could actually perceive everything that's truly going on around you, you'd probably go insane from sensory overload.

And not just "tangible" things like the sound from a dog whistle. "Intangible" energies of the universe (many of which match the frequency of the things you want) are also literally swirling together right now -- JUST outside the boundaries of physical reality (and your physical senses) -- ready to materialize the moment there's enough momentum.

You can't see them yet. You can't feel them yet. You aren't experiencing them yet. But they're there. Or should I say - they're HERE. With you. Right now. They're all vibrationally where you are the MOMENT you "ask" for them (i.e. think about them).

And each one begins sending out a 'beacon' the second you "ask" -- persistently reaching out to magnetize itself to anything that vibrationally matches the same frequency.

You wouldn't be entirely wrong if you viewed these "thoughts" as conscious beings in their own right whose mission in life is finding something that matches their vibration in your time and space reality so that they can "stick" to it and physically manifest.

You're going to use the techniques in this book to match the signals of those things that you want. And in case you're feeling a bit intimidated and are wondering how you're going to do this, remember -- it's way simpler than you think it is. The act of doing the techniques themselves will handle everything for you without you having to consciously make it happen.

You're a bit like a radio in this way. You can only broadcast one station at a time, but you have access to every station out there.

And once you're on the station that you need to be, the music plays all by itself for you.

Now when we're talking about an ACTUAL radio, it's simply about placing your hand on the dial and turning it to the other frequencies. But when it comes to manifesting what you want through the Law of Attraction, shifting into the frequency of what you want is technically just as easy and just as simple.

You only think it's difficult because you're not used to doing it yet. So you worry that you don't know HOW to do it, and you then wrongly assume it can't be done for you.

But rest assured that the dial on your radio can always be turned. All you have to worry about is deciding where to put your focus (which the techniques will take care of for you) AND remember that your point of power is always NOW.

Everything You Want Is Happening Right Now!

Have you ever noticed how time can seem to go really fast when you're enjoying yourself ...or really slow when you're miserable?

20 minutes of getting a massage are always going to seem shorter than 20 minutes of dental work. And if you can perceive any difference in how long each of those events seems to take, then that's proof on at least some level that time is actually just a mental construct in your mind. And rather than there being a past, a present, and a future -- time itself is really only a reflection of an ever-present ongoing moment of NOW.

This idea may seem a bit 'out there' and tough to grasp, but ask yourself how you think you'd react to being told the earth is round if you had spent your entire life up until now believing it was flat.

Are you really able to hop into a space shuttle right now and prove the answer one way or another? Do you have the money, the willingness, or even the military clearance to do that? ...OR do you just have to take it on faith and trust that this really is how it is?

You've got to be willing to see things in a new way without panicking (the next chapter will help a lot with this, by the way).

This notion that Everything is happening 'now' is important because your consciousness is literally rearranging subatomic particles (which determine what you experience in your time and space reality) based on your vibrational setpoint. And your setpoint is determined by your focus. And you can only control what you focus on NOW in the present moment.

In other words, your power to change your life and create your reality is always (and only) "NOW." You're not "hopefully" creating your future – it's already here! It's just a matter of needing to tune into the right frequency in order to have the experience of it. But whether you're tuned in or not, it's still all here happening right now.

If this isn't entirely clear for any reason, don't worry -- it doesn't need to be clear in order for the techniques in this book to work. And the instructions for them will be very simple to use. Just know that you have access to a lot more power than you'll ever realize. In fact, technically, on a certain level, you have access to EVERYTHING.

Because everything is energy, including you. And here's an important little fact about energy that you may not have considered before now...

Energy cannot be created or destroyed.

All you can really do at any moment is transform it.

But it's all here, and it always will be. Which means...

Everything that could EVER exist already DOES ...in this present moment of NOW.

It may not currently be in the manifested form of that car you've been wanting ...or the love of your life ...or the promotion you've been going after -- but it still all energetically exists. It's still all "here" waiting for you in the potential, ready to be pulled into reality through your point of attraction. And that means...

Everything you want also ALREADY exists!

Every desire you've ever had already exists RIGHT NOW. This isn't some wacky claim. This is SCIENCE. This is LAW. And experiencing what you want simply then becomes a question of using the right techniques to energetically line up with it and manifest it. Simple as that. But it's all still just an energy construct.

Thoughts are an energy construct.

"Time" is an energy construct.

Money is an energy construct.

Reality is an energy construct.

EVERYTHING is an energy construct.

Your raise at work, your car, your new boyfriend or girlfriend, your new book deal, your new contract, your new apartment, your new house, your improved health -- it's all just energy. And it's all connected. Your whole life, you've been conditioned to believe that everything you want is "out there" ...somewhere else ...at another point in time.

And ironically, it's your belief in this "separation" from what you want that reinforces the reality that you don't have it yet. This includes your certainty in the concept of time and getting what you want "in the future" vs. already having it "now." That's why things seem so much harder to get than they should. But there's no such thing as "now" and "later" to the Universe. And there's no such thing as "big" and "small." To the Universe, everything already exists, and manifesting a penny on the street is just as easy as attracting a million-dollar lottery win.

Unfortunately, you've been programmed for so long to see a distinction between "big" and "small" that hearing this information may sound silly or foolish to you. Especially the idea that time isn't really what you think it is.

But again, if any of this is a bit challenging, that's okay. The techniques are still the answer. They don't need you to really get this right away. They don't even need you to grasp this ever. The Universe is so abundant and the techniques are so powerful that you can still have everything you want. In fact, if you realized how heavily the odds are already stacked in your favor, your head would spin.

You Are Literally Swimming In Abundance.
It's All Around You!

Right now, in THIS moment, the Universe is moving through every person and every circumstance to give to you. That's all it wants to do. Countless things are already going well for you, whether you see them or not. Even in moments of struggle, the Universe is holding you up and keeping solutions just close enough for you to reach out and claim them.

Do you ever have to worry if the sun will come up? Do you ever wonder if the earth will continue to spin? Do you ever need to worry that you're going to run out of air or water? Of course not, but how much harder would your life be if you actually had to worry about these kinds of things?

Fortunately, you don't have to worry, and just as your heartbeat is already being taken care of for you, so is that job offer you want that's way closer than you think (and just waiting for you to adjust your radio dial a TINY bit). Remember, this is the same Universe that created this planet, the entire solar system, every star in existence, the birds that sing every morning, the cool breeze on a warm beach, the love of your life, your favorite song, and everything else! There's a vibrational version of your love, your money, your new house, your new car, your health, your prosperity, your success, and anything else you could ever want that exists RIGHT NOW. It's all here right at your fingertips!

Which begs the question ...if you're literally swimming in an energetic pool of abundance ...if everything you've ever desired wants you just as much ...if there are infinite resources at your disposal ...if the Universe loves you and desperately desires to offer you anything and everything you could ever think of...

Why hasn't anything worked out yet?? Why hasn't the Law of Attraction given you what you want? Why are you still struggling? What's going on here? What are you missing?

These questions all have the very same (and simple) answer.

And once you understand what has really been holding you back, it will never have any power over you ever again. And you're going to find out exactly what it is in the next chapter ahead...

Chapter 4: The Real Reason It Hasn't Worked for You Yet

Imagine you're learning about the Law of Attraction for the very first time, and someone tells you that you can use it to unlock every desire you've ever had in your life.

You're even given a wonderfully easy 'technique' or 'method' to attract these things. You're then told all you have to do is the very easy work of running through your 'process' every day, and then everything you want will come. Pretty easy, right?

Well if all of this is true and the methods for achieving this really are as easy as you've been told ...then why does manifesting your desires always feel so impossible? Why is it so tough to follow through on this and actually do the techniques every day? Why, when you actually manage to do them, don't they seem to work? And why does it feel like no matter how hard you try, how much you do, or how many techniques you use -- nothing ever seems to happen for you? The answer is your ego.

And when I say "ego," I'm not talking about it in the "overconfident" or "arrogant" sense of the word.

I'm talking about that part of your consciousness where your true identity is rooted. The part of your mind that you use to cope with your surroundings and maintain stability in your life.

You see, even with everything the Universe can do for you, you're still operating on a plane of existence where your beliefs and mindset affect how much you allow into your life.

Which means your solution to all of this needs to include both an understanding of your own psychology AND an approach for how you can use that psychology to your advantage (rather than letting it hold you back).

So what exactly is the ego? It's the part of your mind that rests between your conscious and your subconscious.

3 Minds: The Conscious, The Subconscious, and The Ego

Your conscious mind is everything you're aware (and in control) of. It's the source of your willpower.

Your subconscious mind is just about everything else. And it's exponentially more powerful than any other part of your mind (including the ego). Once your subconscious has determined or accepted something as 'real', it will bring it into your life whether you like it or not.

For example, let's say you want to make a million dollars, and you successfully convince your subconscious that this is now your reality. It will then act as a sort of supercomputer that runs on autopilot to move you into matching circumstances without you even realizing it's happening. Like pulling strings on a puppet.

You'll find yourself coming up with amazing ideas, saying all the right things to all the right people, and making 'guesses' that end up being wildly successful. All because this supercomputer calculated every possible step needed to accomplish this, and then it effortlessly executed the plan through you and your actions. And yes, it IS this powerful!

And it goes deeper than simply controlling your actions. Since it doesn't have the same hangups or insecurities that your conscious mind might have, your subconscious is more intimately connected to the rest of the universal mind. So it can effortlessly send signals to other people who can help you.

For example, it might subconsciously instruct the manager at the bank to give you a loan even if you're not qualified. Or it may subconsciously guide that casting director to view your audition tape AND like it (even if they don't understand why). Or it may do something else that you'll never even be aware of to line up the opportunities that you need to achieve your goal.

Sometimes you won't know exactly WHY or HOW this all works. But you don't need to know in order to enjoy the benefits. The key to all of this is that your ego is stronger than your conscious mind, but not as powerful as your subconscious. And this is why you haven't been able to use the Law of Attraction to manifest your desires yet.

You see, your ego is a survival mechanism. Its ONLY purpose is to make sure you stay alive. Your ego is hard-wired in, it's stubborn as hell, and it knows exactly what it's doing. And it can outlast your conscious willpower no matter how determined you think you are.

It's always going to be more powerful than any conscious impulse you have. And all it knows is that RIGHT NOW -- in this moment -- YOU ARE ALIVE. The way things are -- your money situation, your career, your level of happiness -- even if they're not enjoyable, you're still currently surviving.

And there's no way for your ego to know that you'd stay alive if ANY of these conditions ever changed. THAT'S the problem. Your ego is desperately fearful of change ...because ANY change ...even one that's obviously a positive thing to your conscious mind ...is a threat to the status quo that could potentially result in you no longer being alive. That's how the ego views it.

More money isn't necessarily better for you. Not that the ego thinks this deeply, but for all it knows, becoming rich and famous could result in a psycho stalker going after you and threatening your life.

Sure, being wealthy may be fun, but your ego is not interested in your happiness. It's not even interested in your comfort. All it cares about is your survival. And all it knows is that whatever you've been doing is working (including your habit of struggling to improve your life!). So it's not going to risk allowing any change to your state of being that might lower the odds of your safety.

This was very useful back when everyone lived in caves and had to hunt all their meals. You'd see a tiger, and it was your ego that would override any impulse you may have had to calmly walk over and slap it across the face. It was your ego that made sure you knew when to run, when to hide, when to fight, and when to rest.

Want to know what your ego is thinking RIGHT NOW?

It's pretty much something along the lines of:

"Me alive. Me like being alive. Me want to keep it this way. Me fear change. Change might kill me. Me no like that. Me stop change from happening in any way me can."

Now even though it thinks of things on this very simple level, it's also extremely shrewd when it needs to be. It instinctively knows all of your conscious mind's weaknesses, and it's well-practiced in exploiting them to the point where you rarely even notice it happening. It knows how to use doubt, fear, insecurity, uncertainty, impatience, and confusion to keep you in your place. And it can be deceptively convincing whenever it needs to be.

Think about it -- Why is it that you've probably already learned perfectly good techniques for attracting the life of your dreams, and yet you still haven't been able to really dive in and use them?

What's wrong with these techniques? Are they not fun? Too complicated? Too confusing? Too simple? Too good to be true? Too time consuming? Too inconvenient to fit your lifestyle?

Do you find yourself saying "I'll start using them tomorrow."?

Do you lose your patience when you're doing them?

Do they feel like a chore?

Do they seem unreliable?

Do you struggle to do them daily?

Do you do them daily, but struggle to really focus each time?

Do you doubt they're even working?

Do you get bored with them?

Have you started a technique in the past, actually made some progress, seen early results and then STILL somehow failed to stick with it or ride the momentum to any of your REAL goals?

Does there always seem to be SOMETHING in the way?

Are you reading book after book because you need the "perfect" explanation for how all of this works before you can finally allow yourself to completely commit to it? Does it all feel so ...hopeless?

ALL OF THIS IS YOUR EGO'S ATTEMPT TO KEEP YOU ALIVE.

Notice that you're not consciously in control of any of this. It all just "seems to happen." This is what you're up against. Your ego doesn't understand that the changes you're trying to make are safe. It doesn't understand that some of these changes might even be better for your health and survival. And no matter how much you want it, your willpower will never be enough to overtake the ego's agenda of keeping you alive. Your survival is just too important.

It's like getting in the ring with a 600-pound grizzly bear. You're never going to overpower it.

With all of this in mind, there's one HUGE thing that you really need to understand: Yes, your ego is holding you back ...but that doesn't mean it's your enemy. The truth is, your ego is one of your best friends. It loves you deeply and it only thinks that it's protecting you by keeping you where you are. If you think about the massive effort it exerts to keep you safe, it's really quite miraculous. And by viewing your ego as your friend rather than an enemy, you're going to be able to approach the techniques in this book so much more effectively.

And once you start to manifest what you want and your ego sees how awesome your new level of success is, it will notice that you survived and will then fight tooth and nail on your behalf to keep you from ever slipping back down again (after all, that would be another change -- and we all know how the ego feels about change). This leaves only one question -- how do we overcome the ego in order to do all of this?

Well, just as your conscious mind is no match for your ego ...your ego is just as helpless against your subconscious mind. It doesn't matter what your ego tries -- your subconscious is just way too strong, way too unbeatable, way too unstoppable, and just impossible to outlast or overwhelm. So all you're going to need is an easy and simple way to bypass the ego and set your desired point of attraction directly with your subconscious mind instead. Everything else will take care of itself after that.

Bypassing the Ego

We're going to bypass the ego in two different ways.

One way we're going to do this is probably obvious to you right now: We're going to use the techniques in this book to set our point of attraction directly with the subconscious. They're specifically designed for this exact purpose. As long as you use them, they won't fail.

But the other way we're going to bypass the ego is we're going to soothe it and lower its level of resistance before it has a chance to fight back too hard.

Let's be clear. The subconscious mind is going to win no matter what. But you're not going to enjoy the experience nearly as much if the ego is fighting you every step of the way. So the wisest thing for you to do is to understand this, learn how to easily soothe the ego, and use what you know to your advantage. This will be the topic of the next chapter.

Chapter 5: Paving Your Way to Success

Our game plan for manifesting everything we want in life is now finally starting to take shape.

We've established that one of the main reasons you haven't been able to attract what you want yet is because your ego has been blocking you at every turn, desperately fearing any change in the status quo that you're currently surviving in.

But we've also established that we can get around this by feeding well-placed instructions to our subconscious mind instead ...and letting it overpower any resistance that the ego puts up. So we now have a way to guarantee the results we're looking for. We're in great shape!

But there's still the question of how fast this can all happen for you, and there's also the question of how easy your journey to the life that you want will be.

The easier you can make it on yourself, and the more you actually enjoy the journey to it, the more likely you'll be able to stick with it until you get what you want.

The Skateboard and The Pavement

Imagine yourself on a skateboard. You're at one side of the street, and you want to get to the other end as fast as possible. There's only ONE rule you have to follow: You're not allowed to move forward UNLESS you're actually on the skateboard.

Let's assume that balancing and moving is very easy to do if the ground is smooth enough -- but that in this case, the surface of the pavement is bumpy, uneven, and cracked. This is actually what you're dealing with when it comes to using the Law of

Attraction to access the resources of the Universe and create everything you want.

The other side of the street represents everything you want to attract in your life. The skateboard is your subconscious mind.

And the quality of the pavement's surface is the level of your ego's resistance.

If you went full speed on your way right now, you'd get to the other side. Nothing could stop you. But with how messy that pavement is, you're still going to fall a lot on the way. You might scrape your knee. You might bang your elbow. You might even land on your head a few times. When people "fall down" like this, most of them don't bother to get back on the "skateboard" and keep going. They're just too discouraged to continue. So, they never get to "the other side of the street."

Now that you understand this, what you'd much rather do is smooth out the surface of the pavement FIRST ...and THEN move forward on your board.

Smoothing Through Soothing

You smooth out the surface of the pavement ...by soothing the ego. And you soothe the ego ...by feeling good.

THE SECRET TO SOOTHING THE EGO IS SIMPLY FEELING GOOD. As much as you can, and as often as you can.

Feeling good is the KEY to making sure that whatever manifestation methods you use actually end up working well for you. The more you soothe your ego with good feelings, the safer your ego will naturally feel every day, and the less resistant it will be to any changes you're trying to make in your life. You'll experience less doubt, more confidence, more patience, more comfort, and clearer thinking.

And then the manifestation methods will be even easier to use, which will make them even more effective. And then suddenly everything will be going way more smoothly. Like a skateboard gliding across an even pavement surface. And the beauty of this is that THIS IS HOW IT WAS ALWAYS MEANT TO BE.

Life is supposed to feel good. Life is supposed to be fun. That ride on your skateboard is supposed to be fast, smooth, and easy. Everything that you want in life ...really does want you just as much. Remember, like attracts like, so of course the energies of your desires have that same longing back for you.

This is universal law. And the best part is -- it doesn't matter what you feel good about!

You Can Feel Good About Anything

So if you've been dreaming of a new corvette for the past few years, and that's the first thing you want to finally manifest, you certainly CAN focus on that when using the techniques in this book. But you don't have to only feel good about the corvette in order to get it.

You could just as easily focus on feeling good about the pancakes you had for breakfast last week -- remembering how sweet they tasted, how warm the butter on top of them was, how satisfied you were with each bite -- and the car would still be on its way to you.

Feeling good about ANYTHING puts you in the receiving mode for getting EVERYTHING you want ...as long as you don't then slow it down by thinking contradicting thoughts about the thing that you want. This is important because there are things you've wanted for so long ...that you're way more used to thinking about the LACK of them ...than thinking about actually HAVING them.

So using the corvette for example, if you spend your morning thinking about those pancakes and feeling great, but then spend the rest of the day feeling frustrated because the corvette isn't here yet, you're cancelling out a lot of the momentum you've made on manifesting the car.

Luckily, positive thoughts are WAY more powerful than negative ones. This is really good news since you're most likely not going to be happy ALL the time. All sorts of emotions (including the not-so-enjoyable ones) are perfectly natural, and things happen in life that you're used to reacting to in a certain way.

It's better to let all those emotions process through rather than repressing them. And rather than worrying about them messing up your attraction or vibration, once you notice yourself in a negative emotion, just calmly do whatever you can in that moment to focus back on something else more positive instead.

Fortunately, you can only feel one emotion at a time, so as long as you're feeling good about something, you're NOT feeling bad about anything else.

It really is that simple, so use it to your advantage.

You Need to Make Sure You're Feeling Good for The Right Reasons.

There's only one thing you have to watch out for when you're doing this (and this is actually where most people mess up and push their manifestations away before they ever have the chance to get to them):

If your motive for feeling good is anything other than the good feelings in that moment, you're introducing doubt and resistance without realizing it.

In other words, there's a difference between "feeling good for the sake of feeling good" and "feeling good because you want the good feeling to attract your corvette."

If your motivation for trying to feel good is the corvette itself (or any other manifestation), that means that in that moment -- by 'feeling good' in order to get something in return -- you're affirming to the Universe that you don't have it yet.

Your state of being now includes the 'lack' of the corvette, and your vibrational setpoint in that moment is therefore one of "not having the corvette." This is obviously the last thing that you want.

Now, this doesn't mean you can't focus on the corvette whenever you want. You're still always free to think about it while feeling good. In fact, you really should, because that's one of the best ways to attract it.

But there's a subtle yet HUGE difference between feeling good about the car ...and trying to MAKE yourself feel good in an ATTEMPT to get the car. One is a focus on the car, and the other is a focus on the lack of the car.

Another way to state it is that there's a difference between thinking about the corvette in order to feel good (where feeling good is the goal, so you're actually attracting what you want) ...and trying to feel good in order to get the corvette (where the corvette is the goal, so you're actually attracting the LACK of what you want).

If this seems confusing, frustrating, or complicated in any way, there's great news for you (and get ready for me to sound like a broken record here...):

The manifestation methods in the book, along with the thorough instructions on how to use them, are designed to make sure you're always focused on what you want and

NOT focused on the lack of it -- even when you're thinking about the specific thing you're wanting to attract.

So as long as you use what you learn in this book, you'll never have to concern yourself with any of these little nuances, and everything will take care of itself for you.

But it's still very important for you to be aware of this because you'll still ALSO want to allow yourself to feel good whenever possible during those other times of the day when you're not using any of the techniques. This is where you're going to want to be very kind and patient with yourself. You're used to seeing the world in a certain way and you're used to feeling certain emotions on a daily basis.

On a certain level, you may be addicted to emotions that don't serve you. So if 40% of your thoughts have been negative for the past few years, you're not going to lower that percentage overnight. But THAT'S OKAY.

Again, even if you didn't make ANY improvement on your overall feelings throughout the day, the manifestation methods in this book will still do what they're designed for. You'll simply be on a bumpier pavement for a little bit while you're riding your skateboard to everything you want.

The key here is that you don't have to smooth the pavement all at once. You do it bit by bit. And the less you worry about doing it overnight, the faster it all ends up smoothing out for you.

There Are Very Easy Ways
To Feel Good Whenever You Want.

With all of that said, it's obviously in your best interests to be strategic about this and intentionally insert opportunities throughout the day to feel good. Especially since it's so easy to do. Here are just a few tips to get you started for feeling good in a way that won't introduce doubt or resistance:

1 - Find a thought or memory that always seems to brighten your mood, and make that the default thing you can always go back to whenever you catch yourself feeling worry, concern, frustration, impatience, or any other negative emotion.

2 - Do random acts of kindness. These don't have to be difficult. They don't have to cost you any money. They don't have to be something you don't enjoy. Anything simple will be just fine.

Even telling a stranger that you think the dog that they're walking is adorable counts. Or complimenting someone on something they're wearing - whether you know them or not. Or writing an encouraging or inspiring little note and leaving it in a store for a stranger to stumble on.

Just knowing that whatever you say can brighten their day will bring you genuine feelings of warmth and happiness as well (there's even a technique around this for manifesting money that you'll learn later on).

If you're not sure what to write, here's an easy example of how it might go: *"YOU were meant to find this note to remind you that life is about to get so much better, so don't give up. You're awesome, and things are working out whether you notice them or not. Keep going."*

3 - Watch a funny or positive video. If you like cartoons, watch a cartoon. If you like cute cat videos, watch that. If you like standup comedy, that's another easy option. Watch whatever you think will brighten your day.

4 - Take a walk (in nature, if possible). Just go out and walk around with no other agenda. Calm your breaths as you do it. Notice things around you to appreciate. A couple holding hands is the Universe's reminder to you that this same kind of love is on the way to you. Seeing someone wearing a fancy watch is your reminder that you'll soon be able to easily afford something ten times more expensive. Or if it's more relaxing to

not look around for signs, just give yourself this time to be at ease in the world around you, no matter what else is going on.

Either way, it should be time for you to just enjoy the moment.

5 - Expect good things to happen. But DON'T put a deadline on it. No matter how difficult life is, good things happen anyway, so expecting them to happen is not a ridiculous or unreasonable thing.

As long as you don't feel any resistance while you're doing it, feel free to expect something specific that you want.

But if that's too difficult, just embrace the more general feeling of "something" good being on the way to you.

Because it really is!

6 - Smile. Your body links certain movements and expressions with corresponding emotions and chemicals released by the brain to maintain them. Smiling tells your body that it's happy, which triggers it to release those natural organic chemicals and results in a deeper feeling of ease and contentment.

7 - Write down what you want and focus on WHY you want it. There's a powerful magic in doing this, which will be explored further through the methods in this book. But once you do it, you'll see that it really feels great and even helps build more confidence for inviting the things that you want even faster. More importantly, doing this provides you with a blueprint to base the techniques in this book off of. And that is why the very next chapter is devoted to this specifically.

So turn to the next page and get ready to finally design a life that you truly love.

Chapter 6: Deciding What You Want (For Real, This Time)

If you knew that nothing could stop you, and that failure was impossible, what would you want? This is the question you want to ask yourself right now. And it's time for you to write your answer to this down with clear and vivid detail.

We're now at the point in this book where you actually get to begin creating what you want. And we're only a few short chapters away from diving into the manifestation methods themselves so that you can finally begin to unlock your dreams, attract your desires, and create the life you deserve.

But first, you'll need your own personal 'blueprint' to draw from. What you decide now in this chapter will establish the foundation that everything else is built on.

It may be tempting to put lots of unnecessary pressure on yourself after hearing me say that, so relax. Take a deep breath. Know that there's NO way you can screw this up. Even if you made a list of things you want that didn't have everything on it, you could always go back and add more whenever you wanted.

And if you put things on that you later realize aren't important after all, you can always take them off. All you really want to concern yourself with at this point is what you want to begin attracting into your life RIGHT NOW. Have a clear vision, but don't worry about how it will actually happen for you.

And if you don't know what you want exactly for any reason, that's okay because you at least know that you want to feel good. You want feelings of being loved, of having money, of being healthy, of enjoying life, etc. You can start with just that, and the Universe will have enough to begin attracting things back to you that match it. But you probably have a lot more specific ideas already, so don't be shy. Choose whatever you really want.

You're not being selfish or petty if you put things on your list that are only for you, and nobody else. You're not being shallow if you only add material possessions like nice cars or lavish mansions. And you're not making it harder on yourself by including things that seem way too "big" to figure out how you're going to get them. The 'how' is not your job, and nothing's too big for the Universe.

So go nuts. Write a list of everything you want. And feel free to make it as long as you want. In the end, it's going to serve as a menu of items that you get to choose from for inspiration when you're doing any of the manifestation methods later in this book. The more subjects you have to choose from, the more variety you have to work with. With that said, if you're wondering how many things you should put on it, there's really no right or wrong answer. It all depends on your own personal preference.

Most people usually write anywhere between 5 and 20 things the first time they make their list. Others might have 200. Have at least 5 or 10 if you can, but if there are only 2 or 3 things that you really want, so be it.

Finally, you want to make sure to take this very seriously and get excited! You're about to place an order for anything you want.

By the time you even begin writing it down, it already exists vibrationally (yes, really!), the Universe is already holding it out toward you (yes, really!), and the only thing you need to do in order to 'grab' it is use the manifestation methods in this book (yes!! ...really!!!!). Instructions for this are pretty simple...

Step 1: Add a statement at the top of your list expressing gratitude for all of the things that you want manifesting in your life. You can choose whatever wording feels natural for you, but an easy example that you can use if you'd like is:

"I gratefully welcome all positive experiences and outcomes in my life, including..."

Step 2: List out everything you want, one by one, with as much or as little detail as you'd like. If you're writing extended phrases or even complete sentences, they should all be phrased in the PRESENT tense.

This list serves as a vibrational reflection of you ALREADY having these things NOW (not "some day" in the distant unknown future). After all, you DO have them now (or you're 'getting' them now), even if they haven't "physically" manifested in your reality at this current moment in time and space.

For example:

- "Getting the promotion at work" or "My promotion at work" (either phrase is fine)

- "Meeting my soulmate" / "Meeting the man of my dreams" / "Meeting the woman of my dreams" / "Having my soulmate in my life" / "My loving partner"

- "Enjoying perfect health" / "Enjoying a return to perfect health" / "Healing completely" / "My complete health" / "My healthy body"

OPTIONAL Step 3: If you want to add a little more fuel to each thing you put on your list, while it's not required, you can easily do this by including the reason why you want it.

Some format options for writing this include:

I gratefully welcome "_____" because "_____"

I'm grateful for "_____" because "_____"

Thank you for "_____" because "_____"

For example: "I'm grateful for my promotion at work because I really love having an even bigger salary, I enjoy doing more for my company, I appreciate the extra recognition it continues to bring me, and I love the direction my career is going in."

"I gratefully welcome a deep and meaningful romantic relationship with someone I love because the feeling of connection I get when I'm in love is so joyful, so exhilarating, and so fulfilling to me. I love cuddling and watching funny movies with my [man/woman/boyfriend/girlfriend/etc], I love having someone to talk about my day with. I love knowing someone is always in my corner and always there for me whenever I need them. I love the feeling of being part of a real team with a true partner who really understands me and always wants to be at my side. And I love the feeling of waking up next to someone who truly loves me every single day."

"Thank you for the improvement of my health because it's so wonderful to be alive, it's so exciting to experience living the fullest life I possibly can, and I appreciate my ease and my comfort more and more every single day, and I'm so happy to have them both."

Notice a few things about those examples: They're all in the present tense. And they're all stated "positively." It's good to say "I'm with someone I love." But it's bad to say "I'm not alone." because the Universe doesn't hear the word "not" and a statement like that is really only reinforcing a vibrational setpoint of being alone. Finally, none of them are worded in a way that implies they're not here yet. You could already have the promotion, be with the love of your life, or enjoy perfect health -- and nothing about those statements would be worded differently. When you write them, you should be saying what you'd actually say if they were already here (because vibrationally, they are). Have yourself in that frame of mind.

Also, the process of writing this down should be a fun and enjoyable experience. You should view it as if you're filling out an order form and the company that you're ordering it from (the Universe) will be delivering it to you right on schedule.

You should NOT be viewing this as an opportunity to complain about all the things you still don't have, wondering why they never came. There should be a relaxed mood of expectation and a sense of gratitude that it already exists and is on the way into physical manifestation.

The ONLY Way This Won't Work... Is By Not Doing It.

This works. You just need to trust the process here. And you should make this list right now. Before turning the page to the next chapter. Don't hesitate. Don't wait until you're done reading this book. Take time out right now to do this. Even just a first draft that only takes you ten minutes or so. Just to have something on paper that's there for you, magnetically pulling in what you want with no further delay.

...did you make your list?

If you did, AWESOME.

And if you didn't yet, that's also fine. That hesitation is simply your ego sneaking in and trying to keep you safe. And if that's what's happening right now, there's a gift for you in this awareness that nobody else has ever offered you before.

Maybe you're just so anxious to move forward and read the rest of the book first. Maybe you like to know what's involved with each of the techniques before creating your 'blueprint'.

Whatever the reason, that's okay -- as long as you're aware that you've consciously chosen to delay this ...and that it's not too late to take a quick minute or two out right now and make your list. Even just a short list of 2 or 3 things (if you make it that short, include a quick sentence for each of why you want them).

Remember, you can't get this list wrong, you're free to redo it any time you like, and your future self is so grateful to you for taking this key step in attracting your desires. It's going to make the manifestation methods so much more effective and easy to use.

...and now that I've given you the gift of this awareness, whether you actually wrote your list by now or not, we're not slowing down one bit. We're pushing straight ahead and are about to explore what it means to truly create a state of being that pulls the things you want into your physical reality...

Chapter 7: Creating the State of Being for Manifesting Your Desires

When people first learn about the Law of Attraction, they often experience a robust mix of emotions including hope, excitement, curiosity, confusion, and even fear.

"How could this really be possible?" they ask themselves.

"Why didn't anyone ever tell me this before??"

"How does this actually even work???"

As we now know, part of what's going on here in the midst of all these crazy feelings is that the ego is in full blown PANIC mode. This may be the first real threat to its existence that it's ever really had to face …and if that's not bad enough, this threat is coming directly from the person it's trying to protect!

So it defaults to its standard strategy of making things much more complicated than they need to be in any way that it can. And one of its favorite ways of accomplishing this is by convincing you that you need to understand all of the mechanics behind universal attraction before you'll believe in it enough to really dive in and make it work for you.

And while making you aware that this is happening is a great way to help you overcome it more easily, the best way to accomplish this is to simply provide you with a clear explanation of how things really work.

This brings us to a key topic we have not discussed yet:

Your STATE OF BEING.

As you already know, when the Universe responds to certain vibrational setpoints that you emit, it does so by pulling in energies that mirror the frequency of those setpoints …which ultimately results in new manifestations in your physical reality.

But what you may not know yet is that what the Universe is REALLY responding to is your state of being. You don't actually attract "what you want" -- you attract "who you are" (in terms of your vibration). It's important to make this distinction because it's easy to view a "vibrational setpoint" or a "point of attraction" as some inanimate object with no real consciousness (which isn't true, by the way).

But if you look at it in a way that recognizes this setpoint as an individually aware extension of life, you start to really understand that YOU are really the one who's been doing this all this time. YOU are your state of being, and therefore, "you" are your point of attraction.

You've literally been engaging the Universe with every single breath. And you've had way more control over everything you experience than your ego has ever allowed you to realize. This is all about who you're BEING ...RIGHT NOW in this moment.

Are you the version of you who has the money or are you the version who still wants it? Are you the version of you who's in a happy and fulfilling relationship or are you the version of you still waiting for your soulmate to come? Are you the version of you who is so ready to finally do this that you made your list from the last chapter ...or did you still find a way to rationalize why you should wait until you're through reading the entire book?

Everything you're 'being' is what's mirrored back to you as the reality that you experience every day. Some of what you mirror you're aware of. Some you aren't.

So while we'll continue to use easily-understandable terms like "vibrational setpoint" and "point of attraction" -- it's strategically vital that you understand that what you're

REALLY accomplishing here through the techniques in this book ...is that you're modifying your state of being in such a way that it's continuously sending out a signal of "having" what you want INSTEAD OF only "wanting" it.

Going From 'I WANT' to 'I HAVE'

As you engage in the manifestation methods available to you, you're BEING (vibrationally, energetically, and emotionally) the person who's graduated from the state of 'wanting' what you want ...to the state of 'having' what you want. A lot of this will be experienced subconsciously, so it's important that you don't put any undue expectations on how you're "supposed to feel" when you've accomplished this. On some level, you still need to DECIDE to have it. You need to intentionally change the channel that you're broadcasting, tune into a new and better frequency, and CHOOSE to go:

- From an unwanted state ...to a wanted one.
- From "I want" to "I have"
- From "I hope" to "I know"
- From "It's coming in the future" to "It's here now"

If your state of being is set to "I wish," then you're constantly emitting a signal to the Universe that what you want isn't here yet.

You need to use the techniques to shift this for yourself. The truth is that the frequency of "no money" exists, but so does the frequency of "lots of money." And you always have access to either one of them.

This is why "I AM" statements are SUPER powerful and SO important. When you say things like "I am happy," "I am abundant," "I am wealthy," "I am healthy," etc. -- you're imprinting an energy within your state of being that the

Universe will clearly recognize and respond to. The words that you put after "I AM" are how you program your reality, and your state of being is literally the key to your success.

The 'trick' for creating a life you love is therefore through deciding on a state of being that will summon your desires, and then deliberately (and easily) entering that state of being on purpose. This is done through choosing thoughts and feelings that create the exact state of being that you know will attract what you want.

We're not worried about our beliefs right now, by the way. Beliefs are incredibly powerful, but nearly impossible to change through willpower alone. That's why we will fly under the radar of our ego instead, and allow our beliefs to change on their own (which they will do) to match up with the state of being that we'll be consistently reinforcing.

This is the work we will be doing (although it won't be "work" once you give yourself a chance to try it out -- It'll be more like ice cream that you get to look forward to without worrying about gaining any weight). Before we begin, though, there's just one more thing we need to cover. We need to set proper expectations so that we don't fall into any traps that will block our progress before we get a chance to really begin. This is the topic of the next chapter...

Chapter 8: What to Expect Before You Begin (3 Key Traps to Watch Out For)

You're just a few pages away from discovering (or rediscovering) the world's most powerful manifestation methods for attracting everything you want.

I included the word 'rediscovering' because it's possible you've learned a version of some of these methods already. It's important to expect this, because if any of these seem familiar, you might incorrectly assume they're just like the version that didn't work when you tried it in the past. And you then might not be willing to give any of these methods an honest try. This, again, is your ego sneaking up and getting the better of you.

If any of these do seem familiar, but they didn't "work" when you tried them, you need to take an honest look at yourself and realize they didn't actually fail.

The truth is you either misunderstood them (due to incomplete explanations) OR your ego made you doubt yourself too much to genuinely try them (and you were unaware the ego even had this kind of influence over you) OR you just didn't stick with any of the techniques long enough to manifest your desired result (because doing them felt more like a chore than like the fun experience they should have been).

The key here is that until you really start getting momentum and seeing signs of actual change in your reality, you need to remember that it's human nature to come up with excuses for not pressing forward and staying on course.

In fact, when you first start doing this and the ego is REALLY looking to rationalize to you why this won't work, there are three really sneaky traps you have to watch out for:

Trap 1 - You try a technique out, and it feels GREAT the very first time. But then you never seem to get that same burst of enjoyment any time after. So you assume the technique has lost its effect.

But what REALLY happened is that your body and mind simply adjusted to your new state of ease and joy faster than you thought it would. So the technique is actually still working exactly as it should without you realizing it.

But the trap that some people fall into is that since they don't experience the same excitement after the first time, they just quit instead, not realizing they were still on the right track.

The truth is that this "high" feeling WILL return on certain days. Maybe even every day. But you can't always anticipate it ahead of time, and you can't force it. So you've just got to stay open to it, knowing that everything is still working.

You'll still feel good each time you do it, by the way. Getting back to our example from the beginning of the book, ice cream still tastes good every single time. You're going to enjoy it no matter what.

It's just that for SOME people, if the taste absolutely amazed them the first time they had it, it might be difficult for it to live up to the hype the next time after because they've built it up too much in their heads.

This may or may not happen to you.

Be ready for it and you'll be fine.

Trap 2 - It doesn't feel amazing on the first try, so you assume you're doing it wrong or that it just doesn't work for you. But what you don't realize is that some people simply need to do it 5 or 10 times BEFORE they really start enjoying it. And it's not that it's an uncomfortable experience in the beginning (remember, ice cream always tastes good). It's just that some people rationalize to themselves that they need to feel some huge initial burst of enthusiasm right away, otherwise it must not be working.

As long as you're doing a technique as instructed, and you feel even slightly good, it's working. But for those who let their ego's doubts creep in on them, they're going to need a genuine reason to motivate them to stick with it anyway and give it an honest chance for a few days (or even weeks).

A later chapter in this book will reveal an easy process that you can put yourself through to uncover a truly compelling reason to stay consistent with the manifestation methods in this book. Until then, just remember that it will feel good right away, and it will definitely feel amazing eventually. Enjoy the ice cream for whatever it is in the meantime.

Trap 3 - The craziest trap of all -- The techniques are super fun right away. AND you start manifesting things almost immediately. Results come. It's all happening! -- Which should not surprise you at all since that's exactly what these methods were designed to do!

...But then, for some strange reason that you can't understand or figure out, you stop doing the techniques before things REALLY get a chance to take off for you.

Here you're finally getting what you want, and it's all finally starting to work out the way you always hoped. But then the ego finds a way to sneak in through the back door when you're not looking and stop you from continuing. Remember, it's more powerful than any conscious effort you could ever make. It can stop you dead in your tracks, especially when it's absolutely terrified of the changes that are starting to unfold.

This is when all of a sudden doubt creeps in, hesitation takes over, and you find yourself rationalizing why it was never REALLY going to work anyway -- even as it's clearly working!

When this happens, you believe the thoughts are coming from you, but it's really your ego behind the wheel, whispering things like, "sure, SOME manifestations are possible. You can find $50 on the street. You can meet someone great at the market and make a date with them. You can get a LITTLE relief with your back pain. You can get that part in the play without having to audition. You can land the top literary agent in your town.

...But you don't REALLY think a million dollars is on the way, do you? You don't really expect to fall in love, do you? You don't really believe your back can feel like it did ten years ago. You don't actually think you'll ever star in a Hollywood blockbuster. You don't really believe you'll become a best-selling author.

...Let's just quit while we're ahead and save ourselves the disappointment."

THIS TRAP, ABOVE ALL OTHERS, IS WHAT YOU REALLY NEED TO WATCH OUT FOR.

The truth is, you're GOING TO SUCCEED using these methods. If you actually work them and stay consistent, FAILURE IS IMPOSSIBLE.

But you still need to remember that your ego loves you and is desperately trying to protect you and it doesn't realize how happy you're going to be once everything starts to work out for you. So you've got to be ready for success to come, but you can't let yourself get complacent when it does. Every new manifestation isn't your cue to stop and rest on your laurels. It's your big flashing neon sign from the Universe screaming that this WORKS, so don't stop now!

The good news is that overcoming all 3 traps is so simple because the solution is always the same: Just keep using any or all of the methods in this book. Any one of them alone will be more than enough to take you where you want to go and help you manifest a life that you love. And now that you're aware of these traps, you'll be able to see self-sabotage from a mile away, so there's no reason to wait any longer. Finally, one last note before moving forward...

Throughout the entire book leading up to now, you've heard nothing but great things about the manifestation methods that wait for you in the pages ahead. So it's natural to assume that their descriptions will blow your mind in some shocking and unexpected way, or that there might be some kind of supernatural quality to them.

But they're really WAY more basic than you might believe. And that's really the point! The conventional ways that they're each explained in are what make them so effective. The whole point is that they're presented in a style that makes them easy to use.

So don't let their simplicity fool you.

The true raw power of these techniques will only be revealed AFTER making the choice to use them with genuine commitment and consistency.

And it all starts with gratitude.

Let's begin.

Chapter 9: Signaling the Universe Through Gratitude

When people first learn about the Law of Attraction and the immense power of their thoughts, their first question is often about how to communicate with the Universe in a way that will guarantee they attract good things instead of bad ones.

And the best answer for accomplishing this always comes down to GRATITUDE.

If the only new habit you ever added to your life was gratitude, you'd already have everything you needed to begin manifesting the life that you love. Thinking about the things you're grateful for each and every day is one of the most powerful practices you can ever do. And if you could only just stop worrying about what isn't here yet, and start appreciating what is, everything in your life would turn around and improve.

Every time you say, "I'm grateful for that." or "I appreciate that." or "I really like that." -- you're moving energy and creating space for more of what you like to be pulled in toward you. It's universal law. This is especially effective because it's impossible to appreciate one thing and worry about something else at the same time. So every second spent in gratitude (of anything at all) is also a moment spent drawing whatever you want toward you, rather than inviting what you don't want instead.

More than most any other positive emotion out there, gratitude is the key to truly manifesting your desires because of the message that feeling automatically broadcasts to the Universe.

You see, when you simply "wish" for something, you're actually pushing it away from you. This is because the act of "wishing" only reaffirms energetically that you don't have it, which then instantly instructs the Universe to keep it away from you. Gratitude, on the other hand, affirms a state of being in which your desire has already been given to you -- which then automatically draws that desire into your manifested physical reality.

If the only thing you did every day was feel grateful more often than you felt any negative emotion at all, everything in your life would improve. Your health, your finances, your relationships -- everything! This paragraph may very well be the most important thing you read in the entire book, so don't just gloss over it.

This is the key to everything!

The best part is that once you have a little practice under your belt, feeling genuine gratitude for even the smallest things in your life becomes very easy (and very enjoyable) to do. And before you know it, you're manifesting things you've waited years for.

This is why gratitude is so powerful. And this is why it's one of the best things to have in your life each and every day.

And since feeling gratitude is such a simple, easy, AND enjoyable thing to do, there's absolutely NO reason why it shouldn't be a daily part of your life.

The Key to Feeling Gratitude

(How to Actually "Do It")

Gratitude is a core human emotion that's very easy to access.

There's no trick to it. If you're worried for any reason that you're not "doing it right", that might just be another case of the ego doing its best to keep things the way they are. But there's no "how" to actually worry about. You just do it.

Even so, if you still need a little more guidance anyway, an easy method for experiencing gratitude is to think of something you have right now that you don't want to lose. And whatever it is - think of the reasons why you want to keep it. ...Whatever those reasons are, it's impossible to consider them without also feeling appreciation for the thing that you're thinking about. You're brought directly into a state of gratitude because you're now recognizing why these things are so valuable to you, why you want them, and therefore, why you're grateful to have them. Simple as that.

Can't think of anything off the top of your head? How about your paycheck. The clothes you're wearing. The roof over your head. The food you eat. Your ability to read this book. A pleasant memory that brings a smile to your face. How about the air in your lungs. The last time someone did a favor for you. The last time you laughed out loud. Your bed that keeps you warm and comfortable every night. Your amazing heart that literally beats NONSTOP to distribute nutrients to other vital organs that are also working tirelessly for you. There's SO MUCH to be grateful for. I barely scratched the surface. I considered writing ten consecutive pages of things to be grateful for in the first draft of this book, but then I remembered how much more fun it's going to be for you to go through the process of gratitude and discover (or really remember) all these wonderful things for yourself.

I do, however, want to remind you that it's also possible to feel gratitude even when you're faced with undesirable circumstances.

For example, it might seem difficult to appreciate where you're living if you dislike your neighbors. But that roof and those walls still keep you warm in the winter, cool in the summer, and dry any time it ever rains. And no matter how much you might not like your job or your boss, that paycheck you're getting is still the reason you get to eat every day. And it's keeping you afloat while you figure out a way to get a better job (which is WAY more possible than you've been allowing yourself to realize until now).

One of the methods you'll read in the next few pages actually leverages the things in your life that don't please you, and shows you how to turn the situation around immediately, experience gratitude that very instant, and finally begin attracting all the things you've ever wanted. Another method will give you the opportunity to attract future events into your life with the same level of certainty that you have for things that are already here.

All of them will be useful. But none will be required. So try them. Test them. Play around with them. Experiment. See which ones feel the best. Do them in a way that fits your schedule. The instructions will be clear and direct, but there's always enough flexibility to modify them in simple ways to make them your own. For example, if it doesn't feel natural to begin a sentence with the words "I'm so happy and grateful now that...", you can begin with "I'm very happy that..." or "I'm thankful that..." or "Thank you for..." or whatever else fits in with how you naturally speak.

The bottomline is that these are powerful in a way that I could never describe in just words. So dive in. And have fun.

Your first manifestation method is on the very next page!

Chapter 10: The Stacking Method

The Gratitude Stacking Method for manifesting your desires is as simple and direct as they come. It's also a great exercise to do if you don't have a lot of time.

Step 1: Write out a list of things you're grateful for.

Step 2: Read through each item on your list.

Step 3: As you're reading them -- one at a time -- take 20-60 seconds (however long you personally prefer) to really feel the gratitude of whatever you're describing.

Feel free to write down anything that gives you a feeling of gratitude. It can be a material possession that you own. It could be an event that you enjoyed. It could be a fun memory of someone or something. Let your imagination soar and add anything that you're inspired to.

When you go through each "item" on your list, say it out loud if you're alone. But if you're in a public place, and you don't want to attract unwanted attention, you can just read it in your head instead.

As for how long this should take you, it's really up to you since you decide how big you want your list to be. You might have 10 things, or just 5, or if you're really in a rush -- you might only write 3 things that day.

Whatever you put down, you can list things that have happened in the past, things you have now, or even things that you wish to have in the future.

Regardless of "when" each thing occurred, it should always be phrased in the PRESENT tense (even future events), and begin with wording similar to:

"Thank you for..."

"I'm so happy and grateful for…"

"I'm so happy and grateful now that…"

"I'm so thankful now that…"

"I'm so excited now that…"

"I'm grateful for…"

It's called the 'stacking' method because you're stacking a bunch of things on top of one another in one big list of gratitude. The name also invites you to write larger lists when you have the time for them since a list with more items helps you get more momentum each time you do a session. The more you pile on, the better you feel.

The purpose of this method is simple: Regardless of whether your list is big or small, this serves as an easy way to guarantee you at least do SOMETHING every day to express gratitude and raise your vibration without it feeling inconvenient or being too time-consuming.

After all, ANYONE can take 60 seconds out to write a few things they're grateful for no matter how busy their schedule is. But ten minutes is even better if they can spare it. And since you get to decide how many things you're going to write, you can be as thorough as you want to without it feeling rushed.

After you give yourself enough practice with this, you'll begin to experience deeper and more profound feelings of gratitude.

You won't have to 'force' them (nor should you ever try to).

They'll just come.

When you do begin to experience it more deeply, it may feel like a warm buzzing in your solar plexus. Or it may feel like you're taking easier calmer breaths. Or your skin might tingle a little. Or you might simply notice yourself experiencing a moment of peace and tranquility.

There's no "one" way that it might happen, there's no one way it HAS to happen, and there's no way to predict how you'll specifically experience it for yourself. So don't worry about getting yourself up to some pre-established "level" of gratitude in order for things to begin manifesting. Just know that the method is working (it is!).

Give it a try next time you have a few minutes to add some gratitude to your day, and have fun.

And yes, it's THAT simple.

Chapter 11: The Time-Lapse Method

This method is basically a gratitude "stack" that includes the same number of past, present, and future things -- but all jumbled in a random order so that the future ones aren't all at the end of the list.

This is one of the very first techniques I teach anyone who's looking to make dramatic changes in their life without any struggle, stress, or confusion. Not only is it extremely simple to use, but once you give yourself a few sessions to really test it out, you'll see that it can be really fun as well.

The most amazing thing about the Time-Lapse Method is how easily it magnetizes your vibrational setpoint for things you want that haven't occurred yet. It does this by taking the same certainty and confidence you have for things that have already happened for you (or are currently happening for you now), and directly applies that identical certainty and confidence to future events as well.

You're technically doing this to your 'vibration' and not your actual state of belief since, as I noted earlier in this book, it's WAY easier to instantly alter your vibration (or state of being) moment by moment.

But the beauty of this is that over a period of time, your beliefs will also eventually adjust to your new desired reality on their own without you having to force them to.

Your best bet for getting the most out of this exercise is to make sure you're stacking at least 15 different things that you're grateful for. Begin by writing a list of:

- At least 5 "things" you've had in your past

- At least 5 "things" you have in your present
- At least 5 "things" you want to have in your future.

A "thing" could be a physical object, a goal you achieved (or want to achieve), an event you experienced (or want to experience), or anything else positive that has happened in your life (or will happen). Regardless of whether they're past events, current events, or future events -- for each of them, use statements that express gratitude in the PRESENT tense.

For example:

"Thank you for..."

"I'm so happy and grateful for..."

"I'm so happy and grateful now that..."

"I'm so thankful now that..."

"I'm so grateful for..."

Once your list is complete, mix it up so that it's not in chronological order anymore. For example:

1. Present thing/event

2. Past thing/event

3. Future thing/event

4. Present thing/event

5. Past thing/event

6. Present thing/event

7. Future thing/event

8. Future thing/event

9. Past thing/event

10. Future thing/event

11. Present thing/event

12. Past thing/event

13. Past thing/event

14. Future thing/event

15. Present thing/event

Once your list is ready, read through every item one at a time (out loud if you're alone, or in your head if you're in public). As you go through each, take 20-60 seconds (however long you personally prefer) to really feel the gratitude of whatever you're describing.

To give you a little more clarity on this, let's say for example:

-you CURRENTLY are making $90,000 per year

-you FOUND your perfect apartment 3 years ago, and you're still happy living there

-you WANT TO be promoted to Vice President of the company you work for

-you CURRENTLY are in a happy committed relationship

In this situation, if you're using the sample order as above, the first four statements on your gratitude list might be stated in the following way (all present tense):

1- "I'm so happy and grateful to be making $90,000 a year."

2- "Thank you for the perfect apartment I found that I'm still happily living in."

3- "I'm so grateful for my promotion to Vice President of my company."

4- "I'm so happy and grateful that I'm in such a happy and committed relationship."

This may seem simple, but it is VERY, VERY POWERFUL.

The reason this method is so effective is because most of what's on your list are things that have already manifested in your actual reality. So when you go through those past and present manifestations, there's a "certainty" in your vibration that carries over and applies to the 'future' statements as well.

It's simply easier and more natural for your body to regulate your emotions by not letting them stray too far from one another in such a brief period of time without an external stimuli triggering them.

So now, rather than having to worry about reprogramming your beliefs in order to get what you want (which many people find extremely difficult), you'll instead be using a very simple (and easy) technique to set your vibration up as if you already do believe that what you want is yours!

This signal of "having it" is being transmitted to both your subconscious mind AND the Universe in its entirety without any resistance.

In summary, by jumbling past, present, and future manifestations up, you're basically "tricking" your vibration into setting a more potent and robust point of attraction -- one that you wouldn't be able to do as easily if you were only focusing on future events.

This method is fun, it's easy, and IT WORKS.

And if you want to make it even more powerful, the following chapter will offer easy tips for boosting the effects of these types of gratitude sessions.

Chapter 12: Gratitude Attraction Boosters

While the Stack and Time-Lapse methods are extremely potent on their own, there are also a few fun and easy strategies (or "attraction boosters") that you can use to amplify your feelings of gratitude and shift your vibrational point of attraction even faster.

These are so easy to do that many people automatically add all of them to every gratitude session they do.

(NOTE: It'll probably be obvious, but just in case it isn't, you should expect these boosters to also be useful with other methods that you learn later in this book.)

Boost Option #1: Saying 'Thank You' at the end of your session.

As you're finishing up your list of things that you're grateful for, simply tack on a "thank you, Universe, for giving this to me." at the end of it (or any similar message that makes sense with what you had listed).

You can swap the word "Universe" out with "Infinite Intelligence", "higher self", "inner being", "God", "universal consciousness" ...or anything else that feels right for you and helps amplify the appreciation that you're experiencing in that moment.

Through this extra 'thank you' in advance, you're reaffirming your confidence in what's on the way to you more deeply, which stirs your feelings of positivity even more, and energetically shifts things even further in your favor. If you want to, you can even enhance the experience by visualizing "someone" (or really, some 'being') in front of you to thank.

You might imagine a warm outline of glowing energy in the shape of a human body.

Or you might see a cloud or mist of light. This "being" can be in the room with you or looking down from the stars.

There's no wrong way of doing it as long as it feels good and is amplifying your experience.

Feel free to say "thank you" more than once if it helps. Say it 5 times. 10 times. 100 times. Whatever you prefer. Try it once, and you'll understand how helpful it really is.

Boost Option #2: Saying WHY You're Grateful For Each Thing

As you list each thing that you're grateful for, feel free to include reasons why you're grateful.

It's certainly effective enough to say "I'm so happy and grateful for my new promotion." But you can instantly boost it by going deeper and saying "I'm so happy and grateful for my new promotion because the extra pay is adding so much more comfort to my life, the bigger office with the extra large windows lets so much sunlight in and really keeps me in a good mood, and my new assigned parking space means I no longer need to interrupt what I'm doing every morning to make sure the meter is fed."

If you have the time to include it in your daily routine, this option really helps make every session more robust and enjoyable, and it also helps give you something more to look forward to the next day.

Boost Option #3: Mentally Directing Your Gratitude Out Through Your Heart

As you read through each item in your gratitude list (and as you do Boost Option #1), amplify the power and feeling of your appreciation by imagining your gratitude vibrating outward from the center of your chest as a ray of brilliant warm light. The light can be white, gold, or any bright color that feels good.

This light is your way of offering positivity, love, and even healing energy to the entire Universe around you. You're thanking everything around you for making things better ...by making things better for everything around you. You'll be amazed at how much more thankful you naturally feel as you do this.

All 3 boosters are convenient, effective, and fun. Give them a shot and see for yourself.

Chapter 13: The Blitz Method

Whether you're writing it down, saying it out loud, or even just thinking it in your mind, Gratitude Blitzing is one of the healthiest and most enjoyable ways to raise your vibration, improve your mood, and attract amazing things into your life.

The Blitz Method is simply the process of listing out a large number of different things to be grateful for, one after another, without any breaks. You can do this for either a specific period of time or until your list reaches a specific minimum number of things. This is all about experiencing a nonstop barrage of gratitude and feelings of appreciation that gain momentum, build on themselves with every passing second, and help you achieve a highly attractive and receptive state very quickly and easily. If you base your Blitz on time, you should engage in the process a minimum of 60-90 seconds. But many people have so much fun with this, they often get themselves up to 5 or even 10 minutes at a time with only a little practice. If you base it on a minimum number of "items," you should come up with a list of at least 25-30 things. But lots of people enjoy making even bigger lists of at least 100 different items.

There's lots of ways of doing this effectively. You can choose a specific topic or theme (such as your body, your health, your finances, etc.). Or you can even just list out whatever comes to mind without worrying whether anything you say relates to anything else you've already put down. How easy is it to come up with a list? Just begin and see how far you can go. You'll be pleasantly surprised once you realize you can list ANYTHING as long as you're grateful for it.

You can have gratitude for the air in your lungs, the roof over your head, the clothes on your back, the fact that you eat every day, your access to clean water, your access to warm water, your access to running water, every dollar in your bank account, your most recent paycheck, your strong healthy heart, your arms, your hands, your fingers, your legs, your feet, your toes, your eyes, your ears, your kidneys, your brain, your liver, your skin, every organ that functions perfectly without you having to think about it, your favorite shirt, your favorite shoes, pizza, pancakes, roller coasters, cool autumns, holidays, snowballs, sunny skies, your best friend from the second grade, ice cream, cookies, your favorite song, hot stone massages, your first kiss, your NEXT kiss, a warm hug from someone you love, this paragraph right now, the fact that you can read it, the fact that you can afford to buy this book, birthday cakes, birthday parties, costume parties, the first time you fell in love, the first time you had a crush on someone, the first time someone had a crush on you, the money on the way to you right now, the success you're going to achieve in the next few months, all the people that have been there for you in your life, all the favors they've ever done for you, that smile from a stranger across the room, working electricity, toothpaste, kung fu movies, comic books, professional wrestling, friendly dogs, cotton candy, popcorn, supermarkets, farmers markets, theme parks, apple pie, pumpkin pie, cherry pie, spring breaks, summers at the beach, your first party, funny videos, socks with Star Wars characters on them, your favorite tv show, video games, your favorite cartoon growing up, your first concert, your first car, high speed internet, the last time you smiled, the last time you laughed, the last time you cheered, your phone, your computer, animal crackers, email, refrigerators, cupcakes, cereal boxes with prizes inside, and on and on.

THAT'S how easy it is to list things to be grateful for.

OPTIONAL POWER BOOST: If you want an easy way to amplify this experience, make sure to note WHY you're grateful for each item as you list it out. It takes longer, but it also fires a lot more neurons in your brain. Either way, you can't lose.

At the very end of your blitz, say "thank you!" out loud (or in your head, if you're in public) with as much emotion and appreciation as you can. Say it 3 times ...or even 7 times ...or even 20 times ...or just keep saying it over and over and over and over again for at least one full minute: "Thank you, thank you, thank you, thank you, thank you thank you, Thank You, Thank You, Thank You, Thank You!, Thank You!!, Thank You!!, THANK YOU!, THANK YOU!, THANK YOU!, THANK YOU!!!!, THANK YOU!!!!, THANK YOU!!!!!!!!!!!!!"

By the time you're done, you'll feel amazing! You'll start to remember that there's always something wonderful about your life no matter what is going on. There's always hope. There's always something positive waiting for you just around the corner. The Universe loves you. The Universe is looking out for you. And the Universe already decided a long time ago -- you ARE worthy of every single good thing that has happened and will continue to happen for you in your life. And the Universe is practically begging you to embrace this and allow everything good to flow in. It's all here already, just waiting for you to notice it.

Gratitude Blitz Examples by Topic:

Here are a few quick examples of themes for blitzing:

The Body Blitz: Think of everything about your body that you're grateful for. The huge example a few paragraphs up has plenty of obvious things, but when you really get going with this, you can go even deeper -- be grateful for your strong healthy teeth and jaw which help you consume your food, your amazing digestive system which helps convert the food into vital energy to keep you alive, and your brilliant circulatory system to transport the fuel to every part of your body that needs it.

The Room Blitz: Look around whatever room you're in right now and choose things to be grateful for -- like the fact that you have a roof over your head, the wonderfully sturdy desk to write on, even the pencil you have to write with, the comfortable couch with the soft pillows, the widescreen TV, your reliable laptop, your phone, your tablet, the clothes you're wearing, etc. -- anything in the room is fair game as long as you can feel appreciation for it.

The People Blitz: List important people who are currently in your life (or who used to be), and think why you appreciate them, what they've done for you, what they've taught you, how they've supported you, etc.

The Moment Blitz: Think of great moments in your life that you're grateful for, like your first kiss, meeting your best friend, your prom, how fun your graduation was, that night in 10th grade that all your friends were together and went to the movies, that day your school won the big game and everyone celebrated afterwards, that time you scored perfect on your test, that summer vacation where you got to relax at the pool and play softball every day, or even that first week back after summer vacation seeing all your best friends again.

Whatever version of this method you choose, it's very easy to do, very fast to get through, and very effective for raising your vibration into a much more receptive frequency.

So, give it a try and ENJOY.

Chapter 14: The Discount Trigger Method

I once heard a story of an entrepreneur who was really struggling with his business. His main issue was that a lot of people were asking for refunds on his $50 product, and it really started to eat into his profits. But he was a good man. So anytime someone asked for a refund, they got it immediately.

Then one day, as a gesture of goodwill, he also started offering those refunded customers a $100 discount off his $300 product. He really didn't want to sell it for only $200, but he wanted to find a way to apologize to customers who weren't satisfied with the first product.

And an amazing thing happened. So many people appreciated the gesture that most of them bought (and kept) the bigger product at the $200 price.

He ended up profiting WAY more on customers who requested that first refund than on customers who never even complained at all. From that moment on, every refund he ever processed was accompanied by a discount on something bigger, and he never struggled in his business again.

Everything changed for him because he stumbled onto a way to literally use negative feedback in his business to trigger something more positive. And you can do the same thing when it comes to gratitude.

This works best for "negative" things that keep happening over and over. You can certainly do this for ANY random negative moment you encounter in your life.

But choosing to do this for things that are happening over and over again is easier because when those more predictable things happen, you're already prepared with your specific positive response. So it takes very little effort to do.

The way the method works is simple. For whatever negative thing that keeps happening, have a positive response ready for yourself. This way, the negative thing (that you used to desperately wish to avoid) actually ends up triggering positivity into your life.

EXAMPLE: Let's say you have thin walls in your apartment and obnoxiously noisy neighbors. Maybe they argue a lot. You never know when it's going to happen, but when it does, it lasts nearly 20 minutes and it's a very annoying intrusion in your evening.

With this method, instead of gritting your teeth and just waiting around for them to stop, you can choose to take this as an opportunity that the Universe is giving you to feel gratitude for something.

Be grateful that you have the ability to hear. Be grateful that you're not miserable like they are. Be grateful that as thin as the walls are, you've still got a roof over your head -- with running water, closets for your clothes, a kitchen for preparing food, and windows to let in the sunlight and warm breeze in on beautiful spring days. Be grateful that you can have friends over whenever you want. Be grateful that your apartment is in a location where you can get pizza delivered any time, day or night. Be grateful that you can be as loud as you want to be without feeling guilty -- it's not like they can complain back to you with how much noise they make. Be grateful for every good neighbor you've ever had before these people. Be grateful for the new more polite neighbors who are on the way.

Think of this as the Universe trying to find a funny way to 'scream' at you about how wonderful you really are.

Whatever you choose to focus your attention on in response, ALL of this is taking a "negative" moment and instantly shifting it into a positive opportunity to feel good and invite wonderful things into your life.

ANOTHER EXAMPLE: You have a rude boss who snaps at you 2-3 times a day. Each time this happens, as soon as you have a moment alone, take 2-3 minutes for yourself to feel the gratitude of finding another job at a much higher salary.

Imagine yourself quitting and your shocked boss begging you to stay. Imagine how good it will feel to finally look forward to work each and every day. You're basically using this "negative" event as an opportunity to manifest a way better job with a much better boss paying you a lot more money. The "negative" triggers the "positive."

SAME EXAMPLE, DIFFERENT RESPONSE:

Let's use the same example of the rude boss who snaps at you.

A key point to keep in mind here is that your positive reaction doesn't have to be related to work just because the negative trigger was. Your reaction can be related to ANYTHING positive that you'd like to draw into your life.

Maybe you're looking for love. So as weird as this might seem, every time your boss snaps at you, take 2-3 minutes and imagine being on a great date with someone you're really connecting with. Think about laughing with your date at how ridiculous and melodramatic your boss is sometimes.

This is all lighthearted, not mean-spirited. You're not attacking your boss. You're simply having a good laugh, which is a "real" thing that would normally happen when you're dating someone.

So your visualization is way more vivid. Plus you're now engaging the Universe in a way that's inviting a fun, loving, happy, joyful, cheerful relationship into your life.

The great thing about this method is that if you keep doing this each time, your boss snapping at you will start to feel way less negative. And because of this, you might be shocked to see it happening less and less. But until it starts happening less frequently, you're using it to your advantage and inviting something into your life that will make you happy.

When your back hurts, be grateful for all the times that it didn't bother you, and feel grateful for your body's amazing capacity to heal from anything.

When you miss someone who's no longer with you, think about moments with them that were really special that you'll always have, and be grateful that they were in your life to begin with.

When you're stuck in traffic every morning on your commute to work, be grateful for your car. Or the fact that you have a job to go to. Or the fact that the job is supporting you and people you love. Or for the relationship that's on the way. Or for a pleasant surprise that's coming to you in the next 24 hours. Or anything else that might make you feel good and invite more things that you want.

The possibilities are endless, so test it out for yourself. Give it a few tries to get used to it. Put a reminder for it up as the wallpaper for your phone screen. And see what kind of magic happens.

Chapter 15: Why These Methods Work

One of the biggest reasons (if not THE biggest) that people can't seem to get the Law of Attraction to work for them is impatience.

If they don't see things happening early on, their mind starts to play tricks on them. They ask themselves:

- "Am I doing it wrong?"
- "How do I know if it's happening??"
- "Why isn't this working???"
- "I'm 'Feeling Good' as much as I can! How long am I supposed to do that until it finally works?"
- "Where's my stuff!?"

Here's what you need to remember, especially in the beginning:

LACK OF EVIDENCE …IS NOT EVIDENCE OF LACK.

Just because you don't "see" it yet doesn't mean it isn't happening already. In fact, your body has even demonstrated this for you every single time you've had a minor injury.

When you scrape your knee and it scabs up, for example, do you stare at it night and day screaming "WHEN WILL IT HEAL ALREADY!?"

Of course, you don't. Because you realize that the skin is healing underneath. You know it's happening. You know it's going to take as long as it's going to take.

And if you lose your patience and pick the scab, you'll only slow things down and possibly leave yourself with an unnecessary scar.

This is important because a scar on your knee is certainly something you can live with. But when you think about it, a scar is an indication of something that never healed all the way. It's incomplete.

"Picking at the scab" of your desire keeps it from completing its way into your manifested reality. Losing your patience, letting doubt and uncertainty creep in, and quitting before the scab is ready to fall off is the reason things aren't happening for you.

In a way, you're expecting the "scab" to always be there since it's there now, and your need to control reality and fix this somehow is what introduces the resistance that keeps you from actually changing what's possible.

In other words ...YOU CAN'T BASE YOUR FUTURE EXPECTATIONS OFF YOUR PRESENT CIRCUMSTANCES.

These "expectations" you have about yourself, your career, your love life, your finances, your health, and every other aspect of your life ...are all based on an illusion.

You think that what you 'see' right now in your life is all that there is, not realizing that there's a better possibility -- vibrating at a slightly different frequency RIGHT NOW -- that can pop into your physical reality with only just a minor shift in the signal that you're broadcasting. And it's the manifestation methods in this book which help you consciously choose that preferred signal.

There's another reality just waiting for you, WAY closer than you could ever consciously realize. And all it requires is that you do even just one of these methods consistently.

Now you might turn around and say that a scab is different because you don't actually have to do anything for it to heal (vs. "having to do" these methods every single day). But in the scab example, the "you" that's doing something is your body!

Your body relentlessly sticks to the process of healing underneath the scab, never doubting its ability, never doubting the result, just sticking with it for as long as is needed to get the job done WITHOUT stopping a million times a day to ask "where's my stuff??" Your body commits to the process, knowing it will work.

There's an unbreakable level of confidence and ease because there's no doubt about whether it's really going to work. And just as white blood cells respond to your body's "ask" for healing, the Universe (through the Law of Attraction) responds to the instructions you send through the gratitude techniques you've learned so far AND the other related manifestation methods to follow.

Just as proteins and other necessary components are pulled in to heal the scab ...people, circumstances, and other situations are pulled in to materialize your desires.

These are the things that happen when you stick with the methods and just relax and let go long enough for the Universe to do its part in the process.

With that said, human nature tells us that there's always going to be a level of impatience (and even curiosity) that your ego can leverage to take you out of the game before you make any real headway.

But in response to this, the Universe will find a way to give you enough clues and indicators to keep you motivated and in the game long enough for real results to occur. You've just got to be on the lookout for these signs, which often take the form of small wins related to what you want.

This is crucial because most people can't stick to something for even 30 days without losing steam, getting discouraged, or outright quitting. They need a reason to stay in it.

More importantly, they need to make sure they're actually having fun. Just "going through the motions" of doing something for 30 days without any genuine enthusiasm is almost as bad as not doing it at all. Because, technically, if you're not letting yourself enjoy it and you're not looking forward to doing it every day, it really means that you still view it as nothing more than an inconvenient chore.

And if you have that mindset, you're in a state of being of "lack" that's pushing everything you want away from you, whether you realize it or not. You have to have fun. You have to appreciate progress in any little form that it comes. And you have to be able to identify it when it's here. This is where the concept of "manifestational raindrops" comes in.

The Calm Before The Storm
Always Includes a Few Raindrops.

Depending on your goal -- whether it's five hours, five weeks, or even five years, there's always going to be a bit of a gestation period before what you want pops into your position in time and space.

But that doesn't mean you won't see it coming.

Think about a time when you were outside and it started to rain. Remember how subtle it was at the very beginning.

At first, you felt a very faint sensation on your skin as tiny little droplets of water began pinging your body. A drop here, a drop there. You couldn't even see them on your skin right away - they were only showing up on the fabric of your clothing.

Then the droplets started turning into drops, the sensation of the water became way more pronounced and obvious, and all of a sudden you could hear the rain begin hitting the ground more and more, louder and louder, until finally you were smack dab in the middle of a full blown torrential downpour.

And before you knew it, you were absolutely soaked.

Here's the message you need to hear in all of this:

If you were to step back and take a wide enough view of the situation, the moment those microscopic specks of moisture began tingling the small hairs on your skin, the storm was already inevitable.

Nothing was going to stop it.

You receive manifestational indicators (or raindrops) in this same way more than you'll ever realize. And your recognition, acknowledgement, and appreciation of these raindrops will simultaneously remove lingering resistance, boost your enthusiasm, and speed up the materialization of your desired outcome.

You can't always control your patience, but you can compensate for that struggle by using these indicators as excuses to engage more in the methods, have more fun, and make each experience way more vivid.

In other words, you should be celebrating every little win on your way to the things that you really want.

These little wins are manifestations in and of themselves. They serve as an indication that more is on the way, but they're also their own unique event that you helped create and attract!

Understanding this is the key to everything.

Think of finding a penny on the street a day after you begin using these techniques. One little penny isn't going to make you any richer, but that's not the point. Losing one pound doesn't matter much either when you want to lose 70. But the penny or the pound or whatever else might come -- this is your raindrop that the Universe is using to tell you "IT'S WORKING -- KEEP GOING!"

Don't you realize now that gratitude for even a penny is gratitude for the energy of money? Isn't that all that's needed to send the signal to the Universe that says "I have money!" ...which then triggers the Universe to mirror and expand on that idea for you? Would you be willing to recognize that something as small as finding a penny on the street is more than just the penny itself? Would you be willing to use it as an excuse to smile, to celebrate, to get excited, to be grateful, to enjoy this moment in your life RIGHT NOW?

This penny is a clear message from the Universe that not only does it WANT to give to you freely ...it's already doing it!

It does it with the penny you find on the street, the free snacks at work, the friendly customer who leaves behind a bigger tip, the cashier who accepts the expired coupon, the high-fives from everyone in the bar when your favorite team scores, the sale on jeans just when you need to buy a new pair, the compliment from your boss on the great job you did, the sun shining brightly and nourishing the trees which gift you an endless free and steady supply of oxygen, the loving and persistent beating of your own heart to keep you alive, and the countless other examples that are happening right here right now always and every day!

When you want a deep and meaningful romantic relationship, that smile from a stranger across the room is a raindrop. Getting their phone number is a raindrop. The funny story your date tells you that sets the entire night off on the right foot is a raindrop. The first time you hold hands, the first time you kiss, the perfect song coming on for you to dance to, the feelings of anticipation for seeing them again -- these are all raindrops. Some are bigger than others. Some are more obvious than others.

In the beginning, it will be tempting to focus on other things instead. You're more used to looking at the reasons why something can't happen than the reasons why it already is. But in the end, you can either focus on what you want and bring that about -- or you can focus on what you don't want and stay where you are right now. Bottom line -- If you want to make it through the storm, you've got to be willing to dance in the rain. And believe me -- whether or not you feel it on your skin yet -- the rain is already here.

Chapter 16: The Pennies to Millions Method

By understanding how the Law of Attraction works, anyone with an open mind can manifest financial abundance using a single penny. Remember, your focus creates your reality. Which means the best way to bring financial abundance into your life …is to simply find easy ways of noticing it more.

And that goes for ANY form of money, no matter how "big" or "small" it is (remember, there's no such thing as big or small to the Universe). Whether it's a penny, a quarter, or a $100 bill, money is money. The energy is all the same. And pennies are everywhere!

So you can turn every time you find one on the ground into an opportunity to magnify more money. The way you do this is simple. Unlike the Universe, you still see things as "big vs. small", "fast vs. slow", and "easy vs. hard." So rather than taking on the more difficult task of intending HUGE sums of money every day, simply intend to manifest at least one penny on the ground (which for you, is obviously a super easy thing to attract) instead. And then go about your day. Don't nervously look around for it, trying to force it to appear. Instead, simply remind yourself that it may show up at any moment in any place, be open to seeing it anywhere, and feel the feelings of how fun it will be to find the penny, knowing YOU created this moment through your own vibrational point of attraction.

Here's the key to this - Most likely that same day, you're going to find a penny on the ground. And when you do, this is your perfect opportunity to acknowledge the moment for what it really is: the Universe confirming that this works, giving you free money, and reminding you that there's PLENTY more on the way!

So every time you find a penny, pick it up and celebrate it as if you've just been handed a winning lottery ticket or a $100 bill. Thank the Universe right then and there. In your head (or even out loud) say, "Thank you, Universe, for this fun reminder of your infinite abundance. Thank you for reminding me that anything is possible, that I'm loved, that I'm worthy, and that there's way more money to come. I recognize that it's just as easy to manifest $100. It's just as easy to manifest $1,000. And it's just as easy to manifest enough wealth to last me ten lifetimes. Thank you for all the money you've already been giving me, and thank you for all the boatloads of money you will continue to give me. Thank you."

Or, if that's too much to remember, just say "Thank you, Universe. I'm truly grateful for this and I gladly welcome more."

The point of all of this, just in case it isn't clear, is that you're not celebrating one cent. You're celebrating the reminder that the Universe is always offering you more money, whether you see it on the ground or not. You're celebrating this CLEAR sign that money is always coming to you in massive healthy amounts.

And if you don't see a penny on the ground that day, that's okay, because the Universe will NEVER stop sending you money.

Whenever it shows up, the penny (or nickel or dime or whatever) represents an easy, consistent flow of money to you. One that the Universe is always more than happy to give you.

Your recognition of this and your celebration each time it happens will naturally raise your frequency, help you expect even more with no resistance, and invite the Law of Attraction to work its magic behind the scenes to giving you much, much more.

QUICK SUCCESS STORY:

The first time I did this and opened myself up to finding a penny, a cashier overpaid me in change by two dollars. I snuck it back to her because I didn't want her to get in trouble later when her register didn't balance out ...but I also made sure to acknowledge that I had asked the Universe for one simple penny ...and it offered 200 pennies instead!

Not that you should need or expect something as dramatic to happen for you the first time you do this. Just know that no matter how it appears for you, whether it's a single penny or something else, these are the exact kinds of things that happen when you open your heart and are simply willing to invite them in. And then the sky's the limit!

With that said, there are even more techniques to cover that are way more powerful than you ever might have realized. The next set we dive into will demonstrate what you can do to attract the life you've always wanted with the simple stroke of a pen...

Chapter 17: The Unstoppable Power of Scripting

Could it really be true that you're able to create the future you've always wanted simply by writing it down?

When you do it in a certain way, the answer is YES. And that "certain" way is a manifestation method known as "Scripting."

Of all the powerhouse techniques for attracting what you want into your reality, scripting is without a doubt one of the most underrated of them all. The results you get from really committing to the process will absolutely blow your mind.

Write It Down ...And Watch It Appear.

Scripting is the perfect outlet for expressing, feeling, and leveraging your gratitude. By choosing to script your desires, you engage in the process of "future pacing" -- a visualization exercise where you're imagining yourself as already having what you want in the future ...and then reinforcing that new vibrational setpoint by describing the situation in clear and vivid detail.

You're journaling your future, but you're writing each detail as if you've already attracted what you want. So everything you put down is phrased in the present tense, and every feeling you experience as you do this is even more magnetic as a result.

Whoever you expect to be when what you want manifests ...is the person you'll be describing yourself as. Whatever you expect to have when what you want manifests ...is what you'll describe as having in your possession.

Whatever you expect to do when what you want manifests ...is the action you'll say that you're taking. And most importantly, the feelings you expect to have when what you want manifests ...are the feelings you'll be describing yourself as already having.

You're basically journaling and documenting your day as if you're already living your dream life.

This is one of the absolute BEST manifestation methods that you can do if you have the time for it. And with how good it will feel each time you ease your way into a nice vivid scripting session, it's definitely worth your time!

Tap Into The Power of Everything Around You With The Stroke of a Pen.

It's easy to forget, but you're intimately connected to the rest of the Universe in countless different ways. And your brain is one of the strongest points of that connection. So there are very easy and very effective ways of leveraging its power to draw in what you want even faster.

By using scripting to activate your imagination and create a compelling scene in your mind, you're actually triggering your brain to unconsciously start sending out vibrational signals that will attract the things you want.

We're talking about really potent neural activity here. But because this process leans so heavily on "textbook" psychology, many Law of Attraction students fail to see how powerful it really is.

They forget -- everything is energy. There's as much magic in a standard psychological tactic as there is in any other Law of Attraction concept out there. It's all connected. It all works.

And when you're willing to open your mind -- even if something seems too easy to be as effective as you're told it is -- this is where miracles happen. You see, scientific research tells us that your brain fires the exact same cells when you're performing a physical task ...as the cells it fires when you only IMAGINE it.

In other words, on a certain level - the subconscious part of your brain can't tell the difference between visualizing yourself doing something ...and physically doing it in the real world. It's all 'real' to your subconscious.

So if you keep visualizing yourself achieving a goal, for example, you're sort of creating a "gap" that the mind needs to fill. It's almost as if there's a conflict there -- the mind can't understand how it's experiencing this goal as having been achieved while at the same time still not seeing it in your physical reality.

Your mind hates loose ends, and it won't be able to rest completely until your manifested reality matches your vision. So it works tirelessly in the background to resolve this conflict in all sorts of creative ways.

These include sending you brilliant ideas you never normally would have thought of, giving you boosts of energy when you least expect them, and subconsciously broadcasting the signal of the new desired reality (without you even noticing) in order to cue the Universe to line up similar energies and pull the manifestation closer.

You'll find yourself connecting dots on problems that previously seemed impossible to solve. Or you may come to a sudden realization that there's a better path to what you want.

Or you may realize there's something else you want even more -- something that you were previously too scared to admit to yourself ...because you didn't believe it was possible until now.

These are just a few of the awesome things you can expect when you first use scripting and your brain starts trying to match what's in your head with your current reality.

The Power To Change Your Life Has Been Hiding In Plain Sight This Entire Time.

Scripting is one of the most effective and best-kept Law of Attraction secrets out there. It gets mentioned here and there, but people rarely pick up on how POTENT it really is.

The truth is, your life is the way it is right now because you're telling a story every single day that matches it. You may not realize it, but you're already "scripting" on autopilot (even if you're not actually 'writing' anything).

So the focused process of scripting "with intention" is your opportunity to begin telling a new story for the Universe to manifest for you.

Stop Telling It Like It Is ...And Start Telling It Like You Want It To Be.

Your refusal to tell a new story is the reason you've been keeping all the money, all the success, and all the love away from you this entire time. And allowing yourself to stay in this unconscious pattern will only keep everything you want out of reach indefinitely.

Scripting will help you get past this because it steers your attention (and vibration) away from what you're observing in your current reality, and helps you envision a new and better possibility instead.

Once you've done that, nothing can stop the Universe from delivering everything you've put into your new intentional focus.

Your thoughts can either keep your life as it is ...or they can change it. Scripting helps you make this choice by enforcing a better pattern of thought in your mind and adjusting your vibration to match it.

When you use it to start telling a different (and better) story, you're crafting a fairytale of your own personal choosing and pulling it into your reality simply by writing it all down.

And if you tell your new story for even just a little while, the Universe won't be able to tell if it's your reality or not. It will only recognize your new point of attraction and do its part to begin matching it.

Set Your GPS And Let The Universe Do The Rest.

It's sort of like plugging a location into your car's GPS and letting it do the work of guiding you there. After all, there are always different roads you might take to finally get to your destination (or your desired outcome).

But instead of verbally calling out specific directions for you like your car does, the Universe simply nudges you with gut feelings while orchestrating events in the background, putting people in front of you to help, and moving opportunities and resources around for you to take advantage of.

And if a clear path is laid out for you, but you ignore your instincts and "take a wrong turn," the Universe simply recalculates, devises a new approach, and continues to guide you on your journey toward what you want. Just like a GPS.

Remember, you can only be on one vibrational channel at a time. And scripting is one of the best methods for helping you change the dial from 'lack' to 'abundance' so you can finally start broadcasting a signal that's better for you.

It all sounds too good to be true, which is why most people don't give it an honest try. But it works. And you're never going to know for yourself until you give it a shot. So read through the scripting methods in the pages to follow and choose one to start with. You'll be glad you did.

Chapter 18: The Story Scripting Method

As you begin scripting for the very first time, I want to remind you of an important point from earlier in this book:

What you want ALREADY EXISTS.

Remember, energy is never created or destroyed, and every desire you've ever had is already here. It's just vibrating at a frequency that doesn't match your exact vibrational setpoint...YET.

But through this process, you're going to access and engage your nervous system on multiple levels across multiple dimensions, tuning your consciousness into the frequency of your desired results.

You'll essentially be transforming the energy of what you want and pulling its materialized form into your reality.

This method is called "story scripting" because the word "story" makes it easy to understand the format of what you'll be writing. But you might want to think of it more as your autobiography since "story" might tempt you to view this as something that isn't real.

That's the thing about stories. SOME of them are "made up" for the purposes of entertaining people. But OTHERS are simply a detailed account of things that actually happen in chronological order.

For example, the story of your first day in grade school is just a story. But it's also true, and it really happened.

So for this method, journal your day as if you're already living your dream life. Include details of what you might have, what you might do, and what you might feel if what you wanted was already here.

You can be as general or as specific as you want. You can focus on your overall happiness and describe a bunch of different things now being the way you wanted them to be. Or you could write your journal entry as if one very specific goal that you wanted has now been achieved.

Write It into Existence

There are two main ways of Story Scripting. The first one we're covering is WRITTEN SCRIPTING. Here's how it's done:

Step 1: Begin with a statement of gratitude such as:

"I am so grateful that I make $10,000 every month..."

"I'm so happy with my brand new job..."

"Thank you for the wonderful relationship I'm now in..."

"I'm so thankful that I've met the love of my life..."

"I'm so happy with how my life is right now..."

Step 2: Provide further specific details supporting this statement, all phrased in the present tense.

Note: You can write as much or as little as you'd like. A minimum of one full side of a piece of paper is recommended. But you can write ten or twenty pages if you're really enjoying yourself and your hand isn't cramping. Most people write anywhere from 1 to 5 pages per session.

As for whether this should be handwritten or typed -- writing by hand is generally (and historically) "better" since that's how most people learn to write when they're growing up, and it fires more neurons in their brain as they're doing this. But that approach is only better IF you enjoy it enough to do it consistently.

If your hand cramps up easily or you feel stressed because you can't write fast enough or it feels cumbersome or uncomfortable for any reason -- AND typing would solve these issues -- then type it on your computer instead.

How you feel while you're doing this is always the most important thing, and so the rule of thumb is to do it for as long as you're enjoying it, and no longer than that. This should be something you look forward to AND enjoy every single day.

Step 3: (optional, but recommended) At the end, thank the Universe or any other chosen "higher power" for this manifestation now being your reality.

This is a great way to close out your session and subconsciously instruct the Universe and the Law of Attraction to get to work on this -- especially since, again, what you want is already here anyway.

To help give you a little more clarity on this, here are 3 very short examples of how you might choose to script your desires into reality. Notice how they begin with a statement of gratitude in the present tense, and then they simply expand on that idea. And while you're already aware that you don't have to limit yourself to one theme or idea, it's a good way to do this when you're just starting out.

EXAMPLE 1: "I'm so happy and grateful now that my book is reaching so many readers. I get so excited every time I look up my sales numbers and see so many new orders coming in every day. And the reader feedback I've been getting has just been so incredible. The reviews that are being posted are all either four or five stars, and the emails that readers keep sending me are so heartwarming. It's beyond gratifying to know that all the hard work I put into this book was worth it, and that the words I've written are helping and inspiring so many people. I am so happy that this book is taking off like this. I'm finally a top selling author. I've already reached tens of thousands of people, and I'm well on my way to breaking into the hundreds of thousands threshold. Next stop after that - a million satisfied readers, and I'm enjoying every step of the way as I get there. What a wonderful journey. What a wonderful time in my life. What a wonderful result. Thank you, Universe, for the success, happiness, and fulfillment I get to enjoy every single day!"

EXAMPLE 2: "I'm so grateful now that I'm making $15,000 every month. It's such a wonderful feeling to know that my finances are so well taken care of. All of my old debt is long gone, and I'm now able to pay my bills so easily. The best part is that I'm so good at what I do, and work is always so exciting and fulfilling. I wake up every day with so much enthusiasm, ready to dive into my schedule and take care of things. The best part is I'm surrounded in my work with such amazing genuine people who are really in my corner and who are so easy and fun to work with. I don't even know if I should use the word "work" anymore, because this doesn't feel like work at all. I used to think making $15,000 per month would be difficult, but the more money I make, the easier and more enjoyable it all seems to get. Thank you, Universe, for all the joy and abundance I keep experiencing. I'm so happy to be alive!"

EXAMPLE 3: "I'm so happy and grateful that I've finally found such a great person to be in a relationship with. We're so happy together. We always seem to be on the same page. We love doing all the same things together and we're so excited to see each other every single day. This is the kind of thing I used to read about in books or watch in movies, but until now, I never thought it was possible to experience this in real life. But it's happening. I'm so happy and so inspired by my partner. They're so full of life and energy and warmth and love. It really takes my breath away. I can't wait to see what's ahead for both of us as we continue on this path together. Every day seems to be getting better and better. Thank you, Universe, for bringing such a loving, loyal, sweet, beautiful, warm, engaging, caring, and vibrant person into my life. I'm so happy!"

As you can see, all you're doing is imagining yourself as already being in the situation that you want to experience in the future ...and describing it in clear vivid detail. As you're writing, mentally travel to that moment when this is all happening or has happened for you, and allow yourself to feel whatever feelings you'd experience as a result.

These feelings should come naturally for you, but if you ever have any trouble, you can kickstart the emotional experience by recalling another moment in your life when you were happy in ANY kind of a similar way. You'll essentially be "borrowing" a similar emotion and using it to feed into something fresh and new.

Another way of helping this along is to just put your pen down on the paper and begin writing non-stop, letting whatever details you think of flow out of you. You might have some amazing experiences doing this early on, or they might take some time.

But they'll come in their own time (and faster than you think) as long as you don't force or rush them in any way. Remember, your subconscious mind can't tell the difference between "real" and "imagined," so be intentional, really dive in with this, and suspend your disbelief as much as you can for those few minutes that you're writing this all down. Really "put" yourself there at that point in time and space where you have what you want ...and then simply write how grateful you are now that it has happened.

Describe sights, sounds, smells or any other important senses if they apply in any way to the scenario. If your dream is to sit behind home plate at the World Series, you want to talk about how crisp the crack of the bat sounds when it hits the ball, the raw energy of the crowd that you can feel pulsing through your body, the smell of the ballpark hotdogs, the taste of the beer, the joy of your team winning, and anything else that really imprints the moment into your new point of attraction.

You're doing so much more for yourself than you even realize. You're coding your brain and triggering the Universe to produce the reality that you want for yourself. And the results are now on their way. This brings us to the second version of story scripting: SPOKEN SCRIPTING.

Speak It into Existence

This is basically the exact same process as written scripting.

Only instead of writing it down, you're saying it out loud.

You can say things into a recorder on your phone, out loud to a friend (if you choose to have a partner that you do these exercises with) or just out loud in an empty room.

Whatever makes you the most comfortable.

You can speak for 60 seconds, 5 minutes, or a half hour if you really want to. Most people do it for 1 to 5 minutes, so make one minute the minimum. And remember - you literally have the power to create your reality by speaking it into being. This is no exaggeration. You need only be committed enough to the process and stay consistent in how often you do it. After all, the words you speak are energy just like everything else, and they have their own incredible amount of vibrationally magnetic power. There's a magic to speaking words with conviction. Your subconscious hears you. The Universe hears you. And the Law of Attraction responds. Nothing can stop it.

Script Your Way to Happiness

And Success Every Single Day

Bottomline -- whether you write it down, say it out loud, or alternate between both -- scripting is one of the highest-impact methods out there that you should really do each and every day. Especially since it's so enjoyable once you really give yourself the opportunity to play with it a little. After only a few days of getting used to it, don't be surprised to find yourself looking forward to engaging in this powerful method every single day.

With that said, there's more than one way to script. And the next type to explore is what's known as Statement Scripting...

Chapter 19: The Statement Scripting Method

If you really enjoy the concept of scripting, but would like a version where you only need to focus on ONE very specific idea or feeling, Statement Scripting offers you this option.

Just as with the Story Scripting method, Statement Scripting can be done as either a writing exercise or a spoken one, and the process is pretty straightforward:

Step 1: Choose ONE clear and easily repeatable statement that describes what you want to attract, phrased in the present tense.

Here's a solid list examples, but you should write whatever you want and phrase it however it feels natural for you:

"I'm so happy and grateful I make $10,000 per month."

"I'm so happy and grateful I met my soulmate."

"I'm so happy and grateful I enjoy my work."

"I'm so thankful to be in such wonderful health."

"I easily manifest what I want."

"Money flows to me quickly and easily."

"Large sums of unexpected money come to me every day."

"Large sums of money easily come to me as I earn $20,000 per month"

"I am a magnet for health, wealth, and happiness."

"I am so grateful I'm making millions of dollars by bringing value to millions of people."

"I am grateful for the abundance of money in my life."

"I am grateful for the abundance of love in my life."

"Money easily comes to me in expected and unexpected ways."

"I am surrounded by love, every day in every way."

"I'm a fulfilled and confident millionaire."

"I am a magnet for prosperity, happiness, and abundance."

"I attract love."

"Everywhere I go, good things happen."

"I am worthy of everything I desire."

"I love myself, and I radiate love."

"I am worthy of having money."

"I am attuned to the frequency of love and abundance."

"I attract love and romance into my life easily."

"I trust the Universe to keep bringing good to me every day."

"I am enough."

"I am always enough"

"I easily tap into my inner power."

"I am grateful for my health."

"I am complete."

"I am worthy of love and joy."

"I create my reality."

"I love myself."

"Great opportunities find me easily."

"The Universe conspires to bring me what I want."

Notice that none of these suggestions are phrased in an "I want" or "I wish" form. Instead, they're all coming from the energy of

"I have." Remember, when you script, you're always speaking it from a place of it already existing in your life.

As you write it line by line, you're carrying an energy and mood of "I have this now, it feels awesome, and that's why I'm so grateful."

Step 2: Write the statement over and over again on a sheet of paper (or, if you're doing the spoken version, say it over and over for at least 1-3 minutes with as much emotion as you can without it feeling forced).

You should write (or type) the statement a minimum of 15 times per session, but at least 20 or 30 is even better. Many people don't worry about a specific number, and instead they choose to write the statement line by line until a full side (or both sides) of a sheet of paper is filled. Others write it 55 times for 5 consecutive days in reference to a well-known technique called The 55x5 method. There are numerous explanations, but it all comes down to the fact that 55 times for five days is enough energy, attention, and focus to make a positive impact.

The truth is you can write it as much as you want, but the best strategy is to choose an amount that you can consistently do day after day and build momentum on. It should never feel like a chore.

Step 3: Feel the emotions of having it WHILE you're writing (or saying) it.

As much as you're able to, mentally step into the version of you that already has what you want. Mentally enter this new and improved world. Remember, it ALREADY EXISTS! Emotionally acknowledge (with genuine gratitude) that "this is the way it is now."

Don't simply write or say the words half-heartedly.

This should not be a monotonous or boring process. Be engaged. Focus your attention on what it means to have your manifestation. Feel the energy and excitement of it. Embody it. Own it. It's the conviction behind what you say or write that really pulls the energy in.

Even just a few seconds of this each time you write or say your statement makes a huge difference in making an impression on your subconscious mind, your point of attraction, and the energies being pulled in toward you. When you do this consistently enough day by day, thoughts and feelings of having it will start to stick when you're done writing and carry over throughout the day. You'll feel a sense of ease, confidence and expectation.

Step 4: Thank the Universe for this manifestation, affirm it's yours, let go, and go about the rest of your day with confidence, ease, and gratitude.

The process is working. Everything's on its own schedule, so you can't force it. But you can appreciate it and enjoy your life as much as possible in the meantime.

Remember, your gratitude has a highly-magnetic power to it that influences the Universe in ways that no other emotion can. And it's only bolstered even further when you engage your mind through the written or spoken word while you're feeling it. So be grateful as you do your scripting. Enjoy what's on the way. And enjoy what's here now.

This brings us to our next scripting method...

Chapter 20: The "Why It's So Great" Scripting Method

The "Why It's So Great" Scripting Method is another fun and engaging way to send out the frequency of what you truly want.

The process is simple:

Step 1: Begin by writing or saying a statement, phrased in the present tense, indicating something you specifically want in the future as being here now.

Step 2: Keep writing or speaking to explain exactly why what you've just attracted into your reality is so great.

The format is: "___ is so great because ___."

But you can switch out other words to mix it up. Instead of "great" you might say "awesome" or "fun" or "beautiful" or "fantastic" or anything else that might fit with the vibe of whatever you're talking about.

Step 3: If you want a longer session, pick another new statement and repeat steps 1 and 2 for as long as you like with as many different statements as you like.

At a quick glance, this might seem a little like what you might have done with the Story Scripting Method. But there's a subtle important difference.

In Story Scripting, you were more focused on immersing yourself in a vivid scene, and then feeling the emotions of gratitude for it. This meant one big chunk of information around a specific idea.

"Why It's So Great" is a bit different because you're not specifically 'trying' to paint a picture in your mind (even though you might end up doing that) ...and you're not 'trying' to specifically experience gratitude (even though that will probably also happen). Instead, you're just saying one or two things about why something specific is so great.

You may be inspired to keep writing (and if you do, just roll with it and keep going), but this is more of a stack combined with a blitz where you pump out a bunch of different ideas and you then write or say something really quick about each one before moving on to the next one.

A great example of a typical full (but brief) session might go something along the lines of:

"My new office is so great because the windows are spotless, the shelves are huge, and the glass door lets everyone know I'm around for when they need to talk to me."

"My new car is awesome because of how well it turns at high speeds, how loud the engine purrs, and how comfortable and exciting it is to ride in!"

"The new job is so great because the commute is EASY, the pay is HUGE, and the people are so friendly and great to be around!"

"My laptop is the best because it's got all my preferences set, the keyboard feels great to type on, the battery lasts very long whenever I need it to, and it fits easily in my bag whenever I need to travel."

Bottomline - "Why It's So Great" scripting is simply an easy opportunity to script in a different style and at a different speed with a more relaxed vibe so that you can get into it easily and make the session as long or as short as you want.

For those who worry that they might not enjoy scripting right away (even though they're going to be pleasantly surprised once they give it a shot), "Why It's So Great" Scripting is a GREAT option (no pun intended) to try out first, whether you're doing the written form or the spoken one. It's fun, it's easy, and it's effective.

With that said, all of these scripting methods are solid. But to help you even further with them, the next chapter will provide you with easy guidelines and tips for having better sessions with each type...

Chapter 21: Guidelines and Tips for High-Impact Scripting

Those instructions you just went through were obviously very THOROUGH. So relax, take a quick little breather, and remember that the actual 'practice' of this is super simple.

The robust level of detail and explanation is only here to anticipate questions and make sure they're all answered for you. It's better that you have too much info rather than too little. This is Practical Law of Attraction, after all (wait 'til you see everything I've got for you at the end).

But don't let yourself be overwhelmed by the quantity of the content. If any of it seems a bit full, you'll be pleased to know that when you read any chapter or section for a second time, it'll be WAY easier to consume.

With that said, since Scripting is such a powerful method for attracting the things that you want, I'm choosing to devote one more special chapter to it before moving on to other techniques.

Below are key guidelines and tips that will not only make your scripting a lot more fun, but they'll make it a lot more potent and magnetic as well. Pick and choose any of them that feel right for you.

TIP 1: Choose the feelings you'll want to feel while scripting before you begin. They'll help guide you and give you a direction to go in.

For example, before beginning your scripting session, you can simply ask yourself "How do I want to feel while I'm writing this? What emotions do I want to experience?"

Whatever those emotions are, include them.

So let's say you want to experience pride, relief, and excitement. You can easily put those words into the sentences you write:

"I'm so PROUD now that I've been promoted to CEO of the company."

"It's such a RELIEF every time I look at my bank balance and see all that extra money there for me whenever I need it."

"I'm so EXCITED that I've finally met my soulmate."

It's that easy. And you don't have to use the exact words, by the way. You can mix it up.

For example, if you want to feel "great" but think it's boring to keep using that same word, you can switch it out with a word like "amazing" if it fits in sensibly with whatever you're writing:

After all, "It feels great to know that I'm finally about to get married" doesn't lose any of its power if you say, "It feels amazing to know that I'm finally about to get married" instead.

And "I feel so much joy now that…" is pretty much the same as "It fills me with joy to know that…"

So let your own personality and way of speaking determine what you say and how you say it.

As long as you're scripting the feelings you want to have (or, more importantly, WOULD have) when you're attracting the things that you want, you're in great shape.

TIP 2: Simulate more authentic emotions by writing a letter to a friend.

Imagine that you're writing a letter to someone you know about how great your life is (now that you've manifested what you wanted).

If it's someone you shared your goals with back when you were both younger, reference that in the letter.

If it's something they'd be really proud or excited to hear, write the news in a way that you know would bring a smile to their face.

These are exactly the kinds of details that help make your scripting way more immersive and potent. Use them to your advantage.

NOTE: You can easily modify this in the spoken form by walking around the block in your neighborhood with your phone pressed against your ear, talking into it as if you're on a call with a friend and you're updating them about all the great new things happening in your life.

TIP 3: Write a thank you letter to the Universe.

While it's powerful to thank the Universe at the very end of a scripting session, there's no reason why you can't leverage that same magnetic gratitude throughout the entire session.

Writing something that you know is intended for the Universe from the very beginning will boost your gratitude throughout the entire process. You'll feel appreciation with every word you write since everything you're describing is to the "person" who gave it to you.

TIP 4: Future-Pace the chain of events that will bring you what you want.

You're basically pre-planning the details of your manifestation and describing them as if they've already happened.

You want to make sure to keep this light and fun and be open to the fact that the Universe might end up giving you what you want in a much more enjoyable way than you can think of.

But if you know that you're going to need an extra $50,000 in order for you to be able to afford your new home, there's no reason why you can't describe a few ways that you'll most likely receive that money.

Maybe you'll script about the new promotion and raise you got.

Or the new job.

Or the sales bonus you'll receive.

Or dividends from a stock that you own.

Go wherever your imagination wants to take you.

A great way to approach this is to ask yourself before you begin scripting: "What will it take for me to be able to look back 1 year from now and know that I got that extra $50,000 that I needed?"

NOTE: You don't have to choose a specific goal if you don't want to. You can just as easily widen the target and script about a bunch of things at once by asking a question like: "What will it take for me to look back 1 year from now and say it was the best year of my life so far?"

TIP 5: Include the benefits to yourself and others when scripting about getting what you want.

For example, what value would it offer to those in your life if you had more money? Would you be able to help a loved one pay off their loan. Would you be able to help a family member with their college tuition? How might you better be able to take care of them?

By that same token, what's in it for you? What are you enjoying in your life now that you have the money or love or success or improved health or whatever else you want?

Is there a car you've always wanted that you now bought?

Is there a romantic vacation you always wanted to go on with the right person that you're now coming back from?

Is there a marathon you just entered now that you're healthy and in shape enough to do it?

These kinds of details help answer WHY you want what you want in the first place, which automatically boosts your gratitude, raises your frequency, and amplifies your energetic level of attraction.

TIP 6: Describe your new actions now that you have what you want.

Do you have to go to the mechanic more often now that you have a higher-end luxury car? Are you paying specific credit cards off now that you have the money for them? What are the amounts that you're paying for each?

Do you need to get a haircut more often now that you're in a relationship and you always want to look your best? Do you need to buy new clothes now that you've lost weight and gotten in shape?

Answer these types of questions when you're scripting about specific things you wanted. Remember, this is real life you're pre-paving the way for here. Once you buy that bigger house, you might need to hire a service to help keep it clean. Think about the consequences that you'll be welcoming once you have attracted your desires, and write about all of them with gratitude, joy, and enthusiasm.

TIP 7: Be intentional with every sentence that you script.

Don't just go through the motions and write for the sake of writing. Engage your imagination and see things happening for you in creative and dynamic ways. Just because the physical world has certain rules and limits doesn't mean that the energetic potential just outside of this perceived reality has to carry the same restrictions.

You can choose to visualize the energy transforming in any way that really captures your imagination while you're scripting.

If you're looking to manifest more money, visualize your bank account getting bigger and bigger as you're writing about your new financial status.

Picture the balance on a computer screen and see the numbers start to spin around like what you would see in old registers or slot machines -- and as they spin more and more, notice how the amount is getting bigger and bigger, and how more and more zeroes are popping up on the end.

Or just picture a bank vault devoted to you and see stacks of money piling up more and more until they're pressed tightly up against the walls and the ceiling so that when you finally open the vault door a huge wave of bills comes exploding out all over the room outside of it.

If you're looking for improved health, see your cells as being happy, vibrant, and joyfully dancing around in your body. Picture any dark spots of them becoming light, bright, and radiant. Picture them humming and vibrating with absolute vitality. Literally picture this as you script about how much your health has improved.

If you're looking for a relationship, picture a vibrant beacon of light surrounding your heart and connecting you with the one you love.

Remember, at this point you're scripting as if you're already with them, so this connection isn't something that you're reaching out with and looking for someone. It's something that's already healthy and established with the person who you're now with. Stretching your imagination in ways like these keeps things light, makes them fresh, and gives you something fun to look forward to each time you do them.

Tip 8: Remember you're ALREADY doing it! -- So keep it fun and light.

Whether you use what you're learning in this book or not, you're already scripting every single day. Just look at your texts, read your emails, and pay attention to your words. You're already either inviting your desires in or you're attracting the lack of them.

So you might as well be intentional about it.

And remember -- it's all about feeling good while you do it. So if you're writing something out, and all of a sudden your hand begins to cramp up -- that's fine. Just stand up and speak it instead. Or maybe rather than write down 20 things, you write down only 5 and see how you feel then.

And just to be clear, you don't have to phrase the first sentence with words like "I'm so happy and grateful now that..." if you don't want to. The only thing that matters is that you journal in your own personal style, saying things however YOU say them. There's nothing else you need to do. Just make sure you're enjoying the process, because there's no wrong way to do it.

So don't fall into the trap of thinking there is.

Now that you have everything you need to script at a high level, it's time to give you a new perspective on visualization and introduce even more powerhouse techniques for manifesting everything you want. Turn the page to the next chapter and get ready to boost your vibration even higher.

Chapter 22: The Power (And Simplicity) of Visualization

Think of a blue elephant. Now imagine it pink. Change it to orange. Now transform the elephant into a lion. Hear the lion roar. Go over to comfort it. Don't worry, it's safe. Look down to see you're wearing blue sneakers which tells the lion you're a friend. Stroke its mane. Pet its back. Feel how soft and thick the lion's fur is. It's sitting next to a stack of pizza boxes. They're filled with cotton candy. Smell the cotton candy. Transform the cotton candy into pizza. Grab a slice and have a bite. It has your favorite toppings. Taste how good it is. The lion wants some. Hold out a slice as it gently takes it from you with its mouth.

This is how easy it is to visualize.

Notice how all five of your senses can be engaged. Notice how you can be "inside" of whatever visualization you're having. And notice how it wasn't difficult at all since you weren't trying to be perfect with it. You weren't dependant on any specific outcome, so you weren't under any extra pressure to visualize "correctly." It just happens. I didn't even have to ask you to close your eyes.

I'm making these points because people often put unnecessary pressure on themselves while they're visualizing, trying to "force" what they want to materialize. But "force" only introduces resistance. Yes, you're going to be including "outcomes" in your visualizations. But you need to keep things light and fun and as close as you can to whatever feelings you might have if you were experiencing that outcome right now.

This doesn't mean you have to manufacture extreme joy out of thin air. If you can convincingly feel that, that's great. But it's not necessary for you to get what you want. In the end, no matter how magnificent life is going to "feel" when the things you want begin to materialize, it's still going to be regular real life.

Catching a football in the endzone at a Superbowl as 50,000 people roar with enthusiasm is probably one of the most breathtaking moments one could experience. But the feel of the football's leather surface is just like any regular football you can throw and catch right now. So it's a feeling you have immediate access to in your current reality.

So if you can imagine the roar of the crowd and feel the excitement that goes along with it, by all means DO IT. But if you can only feel "half" the excitement, that's just fine as well. And in the meantime, while you play and tinker with it (WITHOUT getting impatient), you'll notice that visualizing simpler things (like how a football feels in your hands) is very easy to do.

The key to visualizing is choosing something vivid to you that matches (as closely as possible) how it might be in real life. But it's also extremely important to simulate this experience in your mind WITHOUT it feeling like a struggle or a chore.

The beauty of this is that if you've tried out any of the gratitude or scripting techniques yet, you already know you're able to do this easily. That's what's so great about the manifestation methods in this book. They're all related and tied together in some way. When you think about it, they're really all just different versions of THE SAME THING.

Each one is just an exercise you put yourself through that tells the Universe (and your subconscious mind) that you already have what you want and are happy in your life.

The success of your visualizations is based on the quality of them. The quality is based on your creativity. And just in case you're worried that you're not creative enough, the instructions for the techniques in this book have already given you exactly what you need to make them creative for you. While your ego would love to make this difficult for you, it's not as complicated as you might have originally thought.

If something seems simple, basic, or easy -- it's okay. That doesn't mean it isn't creative or effective. And it doesn't mean it isn't more than enough to help you manifest exactly what you want. The Law of Attraction still works the way it always has. Whatever you think about will materialize. So choose what you want, and use the techniques to focus on it. It really is that simple.

See yourself as happy, healthy, successful, abundant, confident, respected, at peace, and loved. If you engage your imagination in this way for long enough, the reality around you WILL begin to change. Remember, your ego likes to fixate on "what is" in order to keep you "safe" where you are. And that's okay. Noticing 'what is' is unavoidable, and worrying that it's holding you back will only create resistance that actually DOES hold you back.

The solution instead is to understand that you're going to notice "what is" every single day whether you like it or not. You just need to be okay with it and use the visualization, gratitude, and scripting methods in this book to set a new preferred vibrational point of attraction.

And as you do this, always keep the following in mind:

1 - Limitations may seem logical, but that doesn't mean they're valid. An airplane stays in the air without flapping its wings. Does that seem logical??? It only seems normal to you because you're used to seeing it. So use your imagination to get yourself "used to seeing" all the things that you want manifest in your life.

2 - Think of your visualizations (or any of the other methods in this book) as an opportunity to have fun and enjoy the moment. Why wait "until" what you want "finally arrives" before enjoying your life? Feel good now using these techniques. This isn't a chore. It's a perk. Nobody ever thinks of watching TV or eating ice cream as an obligation.

3 - Don't let your ego make you wonder if you're "doing it wrong." The only actual way to do it wrong is to not do it at all.

4 - Your focus determines your reality. If you ever feel stuck in a loop and as if nothing ever seems to change, it's because you've been putting most of your focus, energy, and attention on "what is" -- whether you mean to or not. But now that you're aware of this, you have the power to use your imagination and choose a better point of focus. Now you can attract the change you've been looking for. You just have to decide to do it.

You're already way further ahead in the game than you ever realized. And just to help you along even further, the chapter to follow will provide you with a nice varied mix of different manifestation methods that you can play around with and experiment on. Enjoy.

Chapter 23: The Manifestation Method Menu

Any of the methods that you've already been introduced to in this book are more than enough on their own to put you in a frequency of vibration that can manifest whatever you want.

But people naturally tend to enjoy mixing things up and having a little more variety where they can. With that in mind, please enjoy the additional techniques presented in this chapter. Note the title. It's called the Manifestation Method MENU because everything in this book (and in life) is all about choice.

As you're about to find out, this 'menu' will most likely have a 'dish' for any occasion. But please do not let the list of options overwhelm you. While you're welcome to try every last one of them if you really want to, you certainly don't have to.

It's possible you'll want to try everything out. It's even possible you'll want to do a bunch of them every day. But it's more likely that you'll simply want to pick two or three "menu choices" here and there whenever the mood strikes (or when a situation that one of them is perfect for comes up).

This is really the entire point. You get to choose. Go with your favorite item (or items) until you feel the need to try something else off the menu (or in other chapters). Then go back to old favorites whenever you want.

Above all else, your priority here is fun and joy. So read through the menu. Order something off of it. Keep ordering what you like. And let the Universe do the rest.

Bon appetit.

The Mission Accomplished Method

This technique involves combining the elements of visualization, meditation, affirmation, AND gratitude ...all in a condensed time frame of only 1 or 2 minutes.

You can choose to make these sessions longer, but by practicing doing them in a matter of only 60 seconds, this method becomes something you can easily do throughout the day whenever you'd like to easily address a doubt or uncertainty that comes to mind.

Along the lines of the Discount Trigger Method from earlier in this book, if there's something in particular that you're worried about that always seems to intrude on your thoughts throughout the day, you can use those moments as a reminder and opportunity to do this "mission accomplished" experience right then and there, which will then set your point of attraction to a better frequency.

This is named 'mission accomplished' because you're calmly visualizing a specific end result, experience, or way of being -- and then concluding the session with a declaration (which you can say out loud or in your head) that the work of this is now done ...and the manifestation is here.

Step 1: Remove your attention from whatever "problem" you were worried about by closing your eyes, taking 3 deep breaths, and centering yourself.

With each 'in breath' visualize positive white light energy entering your body through the center of your chest.

With each 'out breath' visualize that same positive energy now being shared outwardly with everything around you, stretching as far as it would like in all directions. Relax more and more with each breath.

Inhale (good energy inward) ...exhale (good energy outward, feeling relaxed)

...inhale (in) ...exhale (out, feeling more relaxed)

...inhale (in) ...exhale (out, feeling MOST relaxed).

On that last full breath, breathe in a heart-felt thank you to the Universe for the power it has given you to make the positive change that's about to happen ...and feel yourself completely centered.

Know it to be true.

Step 2: Go to a peaceful and safe place in your mind (like a sunset on a beautiful beach ...or a pine green forest), set your intention for what you want, and affirm that it is now done. Imagine all the energy of existence ...from the core of your being to the furthest reaches of the Universe, and picture it shifting. It doesn't matter how the shifting "looks" -- all that matters is that it's happening.

Maybe it's phasing out into a stream of endless colors and reforming back in a sharper and clearer way. Or maybe it's just swirling around in different patterns. Maybe the energy is now smoother. Maybe it's now brighter or more vivid.

However it looks, the Universe is readjusting itself on a vibrational level to match the new reality you've just intended.

Step 3: Now that the energy has been molded to match what you want -- with your eyes still closed -- give the Universe the instructions and blueprints it needs to materialize your new desired physical reality ...by painting the picture in your mind of what this reality is.

See yourself as the version of you who no longer has the problem you were worried about. Feel the way you would feel. Your desire is now fulfilled. This is the absolute truth of your reality RIGHT NOW. It's happened for you already, and now you're just enjoying the moment in pure gratitude.

Who are you BEING in this moment? How does it feel? Are you with someone specific? Are you doing anything in particular? Is there a place you would go to celebrate your new and improved life?

Capture a snapshot of it in whatever level of vivid detail you want.

Remember, you're no longer looking for the solution. Everything is already solved, your happy ending is here, and all you notice right now is the feeling of profound ease and satisfaction.

Step 4: Affirm this is now officially done for you with a "key phrase" and a "thank you" right after. As you say your phrase, feel the energy of this new reality ripple out into the Universe.

You've summoned the power that literally creates worlds, imprinted a new configuration of the vibrational matrix that surrounds everything, and literally co-created a new version of reality with the Universe.

This ripple of energy can last as little as a few seconds ...or you can choose to milk it even longer -- a full extra minute or two, if you'd like.

Here are some options for your "mission accomplished" phrase in this final step (feel free to pick any one of these that feels right OR choose something that isn't on the list below that works for you personally):

- This is complete.
- This is done.
- It is done.
- It is complete.
- So it is done.

- So be it.
- It is done, so be it, thank you.
- Thank you for this manifestation.

Feel free to try out different phrases. If you're worried you don't have the best one, that's just your ego trying to "protect" you. Your phrase doesn't have to be perfect, it only has to make sense with how you might speak.

The key part is the feeling of gratitude and certainty you experience while you're saying your phrase. You're officially declaring this to now be done. You're claiming it. You're intending it. You've achieved a new version of reality. It's here, and it's just about to pop. You might even want to use the phrase "mission accomplished."

The "Vibrating In Harmony" Method

This is a quick simple grounding exercise that's great for the beginning, middle or end of your day.

Its purpose is to center you and reset your frequency so that you emit a more positive attractive vibration.

Step 1: As you're sitting or standing comfortably, visualize roots connected through the bottom of your feet all the way through the ground to the center of the earth.

These are truly strong roots that hold you in warmth and safety.

If you do this barefoot on grass or soil, it might feel a bit more potent physically, but you can just as easily do this wearing shoes on the top floor of an apartment building and make just as powerful of an impact energetically (there's no such thing as 'separation' to the Universe).

Either way, the roots are strong and the earth is in an exchange of positivity with you.

You are gifting the earth love and light just as much as it is gifting it back to you.

As an additional step (if you want), you can also simultaneously visualize a cord of light stretching through your spine, up through the top of your head out connecting to the brightest most vibrant star in the entire galaxy, as you engage in another exchange of love and light in this direction as well.

Step 2: With yourself firmly and comfortably rooted and supported, breathe in the energy of: love, light, acceptance, forgiveness, warmth, self-love, and self-worth (and anything else that you wish to add to your vibration). You can do this for 10 seconds, 30 seconds, 90 seconds -- even five full minutes if you want. Whatever feels good.

As long as it feels like a perk and not an obligation, you're doing fine. As for what this should look or feel like, that's up to you entirely -- whatever most closely matches the look and feel of the words and ideas you're breathing in. If you can't come up with anything, a white mist or light ball of energy always works as options.

The "Reasons Into Reality" Method

This is a wonderful scripting and visualization exercise for setting a more magnetic and powerful point of attraction.

Do ONE of the following options:

FIRST OPTION: Create a list of at least 10-20 REASONS or benefits to why you want whatever it is that you want.

For example, if you're looking for a general desire of having more wealth and abundance in your life, you might list a new home, a new car, helping a loved one with their bills, or even just the feeling of total financial freedom as reasons for why you want this.

If you're looking to find a romantic partner, you might list reasons like how wonderful it is to wake up next to somebody you love, having a fun partner to go on adventures with, having a date to all the parties you like to go to, having someone to kiss, hold, and love, having someone to play and laugh with as you make your way through a happy and joyful life, or any other similar reasons.

Once your list is done, review it, and reorder it by whatever reasons are most important to you. The reason with the highest priority should be at the top of the list. The writing part really centers your vibration, which automatically makes your point of attraction a lot more potent. And prioritizing it afterwards is a great way of reviewing and reinforcing the energy of each one.

SECOND OPTION: Create a list of at least 10-20 possible WAYS that the Universe can bring your desire to you.

The purpose here is NOT to decide HOW it will happen (leave the part to the Universe). It's more for thinking of possible ways it MIGHT happen as a way of reminding yourself on many levels that there are endless possibilities the Universe has to deliver what you want in this actual time and space reality.

So for money, it's POSSIBLE you can get a promotion, a better job, a winning lottery ticket, win an expensive car you can either keep or trade in for money, etc. For love, it's possible for you to meet your ideal mate walking in the park, arranging a blind date through a friend, matching with them on a website, bumping into each other at the supermarket, grabbing for the same book, grabbing for the same magazine, catching each other's glance while passing on the street, etc.

The truth is that whatever you come up with is only the tip of the iceberg, and the Universe has WAY more options and possibilities for bringing you what you want. Exploring all the ways that you can think of -- while simultaneously acknowledging the many hidden ways you aren't thinking of yet -- is an awesome way to keep your vibration high and invite your desired manifestation to you even faster.

Advanced Reasons Into Reality Method

This advanced option simply means doing both options listed above in the very same session. Do the first option, followed by the second one. If you have the time to do both in one session, it's highly recommended since both options really fuel each other and raise your frequency very easily. Try it for yourself, and you'll see what I mean.

The Moment In Time Method

Imagine a typical day that you might experience when what you want has come into your life. It's only "typical" because whatever wonderful things you're experiencing are now normal everyday events. If you've met all your financial goals, for example, then living in a beautiful beachfront home is really just a standard (but also awesome) day for you. And if you've met the perfect mate, cuddling with them on the couch as you binge watch your favorite show is a regular thing now as well.

This is the frame of mind that you're coming from for this visualization. You want to choose a moment that's really awesome, but also one that the version of you who has what they want would experience on a regular basis.

Choose a 'scene' to run through. It can be anywhere from 90 seconds to 5 minutes or even 10 minutes.

What's happening in this scene? Where are you? Who are you with? What are you wearing? What do you look like? What are you doing? Are you indoors or outdoors? What season is it? Are you relaxing or are you doing an activity? What are the sights, sounds, and smells around you? Are you wearing different clothes than you used to wear? Is your hair styled differently?

What about any of these details are clear indicators that you now have what you want? Play this scene out in your head from your point of view. You're not somewhere floating above this person watching them live this life -- rather, you ARE this person living through this, seeing what they see, hearing what they hear, feeling what they feel. This is you.

Do this meditation for at least 90 seconds. But 5 or 10 minutes is even better. This is also a great visualization to do as you're drifting off to sleep, since this experience will be your last thought of the day and therefore a clear instruction for your subconscious mind (AND the Universe) to begin working towards while you sleep. If you do it right before bed, you might also be pleased to notice that you get to sleep quicker and more easily AND you sleep more soundly throughout the night since you're infusing positive emotions that carry you through into the morning.

The Instant Replay Method

This is another 'end result' visualization where you take a snippet (of only a few seconds) of what it would be like to have what you want ...and replay it in your mind over and over again.

This method is basically a modification of The Moment in Time Method. Only in this visualization, rather than imagining an entire highly-detailed scene, you choose a specific 30-second "clip" and just play that out a few times.

You can even go deeper and choose just 5 seconds that REALLY highlight the moment for you. Just play it over and over again, and really enjoy it.

Maybe focus on the sights of the experience on the first replay, then the sounds on the next, then the smells, the feelings, the sights again, the feelings again, the sights, the feelings, the sounds, etc. Just play it over and over again. Do this for 90 seconds or five minutes or as you're going to bed. The more you play it in your mind, the more real it will feel both consciously and subconsciously, and that's when the magic really starts happening.

The "Ten Minutes Ago" Method

If you can vividly picture yourself in the exact moment when you're getting what you want, that's definitely something you should do. And maybe you're fortunate enough that this kind of thing comes easily for you.

But for many people, it's not so easy, and they often have trouble visualizing those very specific moments. They worry that they're not 'feeling it' enough. Or they struggle to come up with 'exact' or 'perfect' details to have in their visualization. But really, what they do is put way too much pressure on themselves. That's the real reason they seem to have so much difficulty with this. It's all just a false limiting belief.

If you attempt to visualize the exact moment when you're getting something, and you have this same issue, this is most likely more of the ego doing its work behind the scenes trying to keep you "safe." Even so, you still might want to play around and try these kinds of visualizations for 5 minutes, 2 minutes, or even 1 minute without worrying about being perfect (as long as you're not letting yourself get too frustrated). Think of it as experimenting and just playing with it and seeing where it goes. But while you're at it, a great strategy that makes visualizing success MUCH easier for most people is the "Ten Minutes Ago" technique.

The technique is simple: You're visualizing yourself, your feelings, and your surroundings as if you received the news of your manifestation just ten minutes ago.

The brilliance of this is that after you've had ten minutes to 'process' the awesome news you just got, there's no "perfect" emotion you should expect to feel. You MIGHT still be just as excited as the exact moment you got the news. But you also might be way calmer and in a state of relaxed ease and bliss.

However it might possibly play out, you've given yourself this extra bit of distance between when you "received the news" and any potential settling down from that initial rush.

So it helps everything feel way more real to you (and by result, your subconscious). This extra layer of realism fires trillions of extra brain cells to help collapse the overall time it will take for your manifestation to appear in your reality.

The point of this technique is you can pick any emotion along the spectrum that's both believable AND accessible ...because ANY emotion ten minutes later is ALREADY believable ...and whatever level of excitement you feel in that moment is the perfect level for you. After all, by the time ten minutes has passed, the news has now sunk in. Whatever you're thinking or feeling, this is now your reality.

The feeling you have as this new version of you CAN be dramatic, but it doesn't have to be. There's no perfect answer you have to figure out. You've left your ego no backdoors to sneak into to sabotage you here. And if your ego is rationalizing that ten minutes is still too soon, then choose 20. Or an hour. Or a day. Regardless, this technique is just another enjoyable way of "tricking" your vibration into matching up with your desired success.

The "Two Years From Now"
Letter Scripting Method

Picture yourself 2 years in the future finally living your dream life. Imagine what it's like. Imagine who you've become. You're as happy, fulfilled, and successful as you always wanted to be.

Looking back from this vantage point, what would have had to happen in order for you to be living this dream life? Whatever that is, script it out as if you're writing your past self a letter to let them know what they have to look forward to.

Remember to use "I am" and "I have" statements. Keep it all in the present tense. It's either happening right now ("I'm living in the perfect apartment") or it's already happened ("I found the perfect apartment"). Begin some of the sentences with standard gratitude phrases like "I am so grateful now that..."

When you've put yourself in this state of mind and you're writing from this vantage point, it's easy to be excited, grateful, and content.

You still get the benefit of feeling you've succeeded, but because it's a 2-year gap you're writing from, it's also more plausible to your mind that you truly could have accomplished this, so it's more realistic for your brain to accept without any of the baggage of your current limiting beliefs getting in the way. You get to experience what you want without having to force it.

If you don't like the idea of doing this from the vantage point of 2 years, then describe "the past year" instead. Or even the past 6 months. Or any time frame that feels good to you. But I personally recommend you first try it as your future self of at least 2 years from now. You're choosing a minimum of 2 years because if you pick a shorter time frame like only 6 months, your ego might be able to sneak enough doubt in to dilute the effect and weaken your vibrational setpoint. But 2 years is more than enough time to be believable.

And remember, it's not like you had to wait a full 2 years for everything to come. Maybe it only took you a year and a half, and you've been enjoying everything for the past 6 months, and you've simply waited until the 2 year mark to document it back in a letter for your past self. Maybe it took even less time.

The beauty is it could have happened AT ANY POINT in those two years, which keeps things 'soft' enough so that you can just enjoy the feeling of having it now (as the version of you 2 years in the future) without any feelings of doubt or resistance getting in the way or creeping in.

You can script 1 page ...or 3 pages ...or even 5 pages. Whatever feels fun. Whatever doesn't feel like a chore. As long as you're enjoying it, it's doing what it's supposed to.

And if you do this every day (or even every other day), you will be SHOCKED and AMAZED at what happens in your life.

Remember to end your letter on a note of pure gratitude for extra impact. Thank your earlier self for sticking with the techniques.

The "Protecting The Prize" Method

There was a story of a mixed martial artist who wanted to be a world champion in the women's strawweight division of the UFC (Strawweight fighters compete at a weight of 115 lb, and UFC is the biggest promoter of organized professional fights in the world.).

When asked in an interview how she prepares mentally, she mentioned two visualizations that her sports psychologist puts her through.

One is a vivid scene where she's winning the world title.

The other ...is a scenario in which she's defending it.

This second visualization is a brilliant strategy because it's consistently putting her in a mental (and universally energetic) simulation of already having achieved her goal.

It's a profoundly magnetic vibrational setpoint. And doing something like this for just 5 minutes, 3 minutes, or even 90 seconds serves as a wonderfully effective visualization session.

As of this writing, she's already #7 in the world.

Here are two quick examples of how you can apply this for yourself: (Keep in mind, this method uses the word "protecting" because the strawweight fighter 'defending' her championship is such a clear example of how and why this works. But it's not so much about "protecting" what you have as it is "maintaining" or "keeping" it.)

Example 1: "PROTECTING" YOUR MONEY

If you want to make a million dollars, visualizing yourself receiving that money is a great strategy. But an even stronger one is visualizing what you would do once you had the money.

What investments might you make with it? Would you put some of it in real estate? Or bonds? Or somewhere else?

Visualize yourself in meetings with professional money managers or high level accountants having these important conversations about the money that's ALREADY in your account. These conversations should be fun and exciting, not boring.

Example 2: "PROTECTING" YOUR RELATIONSHIP

If you want to be in a healthy loving relationship, visualizing yourself meeting someone special is a great strategy. But an even stronger one is visualizing what you would do once you were in that relationship.

What kind of dates would you plan with this person to keep the romance going? What kind of home would you eventually look for together? What kind of decisions would you need to make as a couple?

Visualize conversations like how you're going to share closet space together (these should be fun discussions, not arguments). Does one of you have a guitar that you need to make room for? Do one or both of you have lots of clothes?

These are real issues to figure out when you're ALREADY WITH somebody special. Engage yourself deeply in this exercise.

KEY TAKEAWAY: If you want to manifest a specific experience, achievement, or thing -- pick a clear and detailed scenario to visualize where you've got it already. Feel what it feels like to be the person who's already achieved what they wanted. BE the person who has it. THAT'S the signal you want to send out to the Universe.

You only ever want something because you believe that having it will feel good. So these visualizations should be awesome experiences.

Whether it's five minutes, or even less (or more if you're REALLY enjoying yourself with them), these are your opportunities to experience joy and fulfillment RIGHT NOW without having to wait another second longer. Enjoy them.

Chapter 24: An Easy Way to Meditate

Like everything else related to the Law of Attraction, people often find a way of overcomplicating meditation and never give themselves the opportunity to really benefit from it. But once you understand what meditation really is and how it best fits in with attracting the things that you want, it often ends up becoming one of the most enjoyable manifestation methods to use.

With that said, there are really only 2 ways I know of for meditating successfully. One is by directing your thoughts and focus in a specific direction (that you choose). The other is having no thought at all and emptying your mind (if you can).

When it comes to emptying your mind, there's no real magic formula. You just practice it until you get good at doing it. It usually isn't something that comes naturally to most people, so it requires patience. And if you really want to meditate in this way, your best bet of having a productive session is to:

- Make sure you're always taking deep calm breaths.

- Stay in quiet environments where you won't be disturbed.

- Accept the fact that -- in the beginning -- thoughts will definitely intrude.

- ...And just patiently and gently let those thoughts go as soon as they come ...until it eventually begins to get easier and easier over time.

OR ...you can do what I like to do, go with the first method, and instead intentionally choose to consciously hold a point of focus during your meditation session. This option is the easiest one for most people, and it's extremely potent and effective.

As for what qualifies as a useful and easy point of focus, there are plenty of options to choose from. You can count your breaths. You can think of a specific image to focus on. You can visualize a scene in your head. You can be in the scene that you're visualizing. The possibilities are endless.

And if any unwanted thoughts intrude, they're way easier to deal with since you're not worried about keeping your mind absolutely silent -- and you can instead just redirect your focus to wherever you want it to be.

Ultimately, when you're doing it right (and it's very easy to do it right), meditation becomes a fun distraction from the rest of your day. And it easily provides enough feelings of ease and joy to help you shift your frequency into a mode of receiving.

With that in mind, the next chapter will provide you with a meditation you can use for relaxing your mind and stimulating your vibration to attract more abundance in your life.

You'll notice right away that it's geared specifically around money, but I'll show you how to modify it for other things like health and relationships toward the end.

Chapter 25: The Ultimate Money Meditation Method

This is great to do first thing in the morning, but you can really do it whenever you like. The purpose of this meditation is to lower stress, increase ease, raise your frequency, and enhance your vibrational signal for inviting in more money.

Find a comfortable position (either sitting or lying down), and take 3 slow easy deep breaths.

Imagine yourself on a beach. The sun is bright and feels wonderful on your skin. The sand is warm and feels cozy between your toes. And the water is the most gorgeous radiant kind of blue you've ever seen in your entire life. It stretches out endlessly past the horizon. Mixed in with the blue are shimmering waves of white and gold.

This water is known as the Endless Ocean of Abundance. Anyone who's willing to go there and receive from it can find it. This is YOUR personal source to the abundance of the Universe. It's for you and you alone.

If you ever want to invite anyone else to join you for any reason, you can. But they always have access to their own ocean, and their presence at yours requires your invitation.

Feel the soothing breeze on your skin, breathe the fresh warm air in, and let the low tide of silky smooth water gently wash across your feet. Say "Thank You" to the Universe for this truly joyful experience.

The ocean in front of you is self-replenishing. It will never run dry. It will never disappear. It is infinite, unlimited, and eternal. And your gratitude nurtures it even further in every single moment. With even just one simple "thank you" or other expression of appreciation, you've given this ocean more than it could ever ask for. And now it wants to give back to you in even higher orders of magnitude.

So bring a cup to the edge of the shore where the sand meets the water. Or bring a bucket. Or a barrel. Or any container of any size that you wish. You can use it as many times as you want while you're there, so it doesn't matter how big or small it is. All that matters is your comfort and your preference.

Let's say you're using a large but light bucket (but choose whatever you want). Let the water flow into the bucket until it's overflowing. Move a few steps back, turn, and pour the water out onto the sand. The blue parts of the water gently return to the ocean, while the white and gold transform in front of you into large piles of cash.

As you empty your bucket on the sand, and cash begins to form -- it multiplies effortlessly into huge stacks on the beach for you. There's a slight breeze, but the stacks of cash are way too big to blow away. Your money's not going anywhere.

These stacks of cash are now yours. Give them permission to float into your bank account and watch as they drift there for you at your command. You can go a few steps back toward the water and get more money now if you want, or you can just wait to do it again tomorrow.

The supply is endless. There's always more than enough. The Universe is unlimited and it WANTS you to have it all. You're invited back to this ocean anytime you want. You're always welcome here.

Before you leave, show your gratitude one more time with a warm genuine "THANK YOU." Allow yourself to feel the feelings of this abundance, this prosperity, this gratitude, this ease, this joy, this wealth, and this love that the Universe always has for you.

Do this every morning (or any part of the day you want) and watch reality mirror abundance back into your life in ways that will take your breath away.

MODIFICATION NOTE: Remember, this is the Endless Ocean of ABUNDANCE. That can mean money, but you can also use this for other things you wish to attract that will add joy to your life. The gold water can transform into health and vitality as you're drinking it in. It can transform into a beacon of light to reach out and energetically summon your perfect romantic partner. Or you can instead treat the water like an elixir that cleans up your vibration for love and removes any barriers around your heart when you drink it.

It can even morph into inspiration for a new book or business idea, and as you visualize yourself massaging your scalp with the water, it gently sinks in and revitalizes your brain, activating its most creative sections. It's your ocean, so you get to make the rules. Have fun with it and enjoy the process.

Chapter 26: The Walking Meditation Method

While there's still some extremely VITAL content to go through in the rest of this book, you're now reading the final featured 'method' in it. And we're ending things on a very high and POWERFULLY effective note.

This technique is one of the best you can do because it's deeply immersive, super fun, and literally takes no extra time out of your day since you'll be doing it during your normal everyday schedule. So you can do this literally anywhere or any time. You can do it on the way to work, on the way home, on the way to a date, sitting in your car stuck in traffic, on an elevator, or literally any place else.

The method is simply to emotionally "step" into the shoes of a version of you who has what you want, embody the energy of that experience, and literally walk through your day as that person while "living" their experience.

The great thing about this technique is that you don't have to go through some deep 2-hour mental exercise in order to successfully do it. You simply view the world in front of you as your stage, step right onto it, and play the part.

You really are an actor of sorts when you're doing this. You're playing the role as convincingly as you can. You're walking like the version of you who has what they want, talking like that version, doing things like that person does, etc. So ask yourself how it feels to be that person. And then embody what you think the answer is. You want your body to begin to feel as if this is really happening. You're giving a brilliant, vivid, convincing, authentic, and dynamic performance.

You're now a walking talking breathing visualization that's come alive in this physical reality.

You literally become the walking embodiment of this new version of you, which energetically tells the Universe that it now needs to match the signal of whatever happiness or success this new you has achieved.

And you're not making this difficult in any way. Remember, it can be as long or as short of an experience as you want it to be. As soon as it feels like a chore (assuming that even happens), stop right then and there. Ultimately, this is about keeping your biochemistry in a happy place and coming from the mindset that you're genuinely making this fun.

So ...have fun with this. Get into character and really play the role as if you're performing for the world, for your subconscious mind, for your ego, and for the entire Universe as well. This should be method acting at its finest. You should be living this on any and every level that inspires you.

You should be walking like the version of you who now has what you want. You should be moving like this version of you. You should be thinking like this version. Have the same healthy attitude and outlook on life as this version. Have the same level of confidence as this version. Literally BE this version. Think intentionally about what your experience really should be here. Ask yourself: Does the 'you' who has what they want move briskly because they're very excited and enthusiastic ...or do they move slowly because they're very much at ease and never in a rush?

Really put yourself in that new version's shoes in everything that you do. Does this version of you run to catch the subway because they're late for work ...or do they not care because they are their own boss? Or maybe they do run, but it's only because they're about to sit front row at the NBA Finals or the World

Series or some other big event, and they're really excited and they don't want to be late. Or maybe they're on their way to a date with their soulmate. Or maybe they're on their way to close on a new home they've just purchased. Whatever they're doing or whatever the reason they may or may not be in a rush, you should feel it as much as you can.

And you should do this if you're actually at a subway or other form of public transportation in real life. If you're driving a car instead, answer questions about the new version of you from that scenario. You're not making up places to go -- you're actually going wherever the current version of you has to be BUT going there AS the version of you that already has what they want. The world is your canvas here, and the possibilities are endless. So really get into it and let it snowball as you do this walking meditation longer and longer and your feelings of fulfillment get bigger, better, fuller and grander.

Walk through the world with the ease that your best self would. And then sit back while the Universe mirrors greater manifestations to you than you ever could have imagined. This concludes the Manifestation Method portion of the book. But there's still more critical content that we really need to cover. Because now that you have all of these powerful and potent techniques under your belt, you really need to seize this opportunity and guarantee yourself a way of making sure you actually use them. The next chapter will take you deeper into this vital conversation.

Chapter 27: Strategies for Sticking with It

You now officially have all the tools you'll ever need at your disposal for setting your point of attraction where you want it to be, unlocking your dreams, and manifesting a life you truly love.

But as you dive in to get started with this, the critical momentum that you build on your journey may or may not always be obvious to you, especially in the beginning.

So in order to make sure you don't lose your way or fall off course, this chapter has been written to offer key strategies for easing into an enjoyable routine to help you stay consistent without allowing doubt or frustration to throw you off track.

In other words, these strategies will be everything you need to gently nudge your ego out of the way any time you normally would have allowed it to stop you in the past.

This is the point where the rubber really meets the road and most people fall short. But for you, this is the moment when things really take off instead.

Here Are 10 Strategies for Staying on Course

And Using These Methods the Way They Were Always Meant to Be Used.

Strategy 1: Expect Excuses

Excuses for NOT doing the manifestation methods in this book are going to come one way or another.

You need to expect them or they'll always have power over you and keep you from doing what you need to. Remember, this is a brand new change you're making to your life.

So until you give yourself the chance to do it for a few days and pick up some steam, your ego is still running the show (even when it doesn't seem like it).

It WILL find a way to rationalize why you shouldn't be doing the techniques no matter how easy, enjoyable, or convenient they are.

But if you expect those excuses to pop up, you'll be ready for them. This all goes back to the workout example at the beginning of this book. Imagine wanting to start a daily routine of going to the gym. You realize it's good for you. You just paid a huge membership fee. And you even know that once you get there and work up a sweat, your body is going to feel great. Seems like there's no real reason to put it off.

But as you wake up that day, you remember you've got an important early meeting. So you skip your morning workout to get ahead of the traffic, thinking you can exercise on your lunch hour instead.

But the meeting goes longer than you expected, your emails are backed up, and someone's breathing down your neck for something they weren't supposed to need until next week. Now you've got to work through lunch. So the new plan is to hit the gym right after work. But as your day comes to a close, you're just way too exhausted to change clothes, drive a few miles out of your way, and push yourself through an hour of treadmills, weights, or whatever else you were supposed to do.

And before you know it, you're getting ready for bed, wondering why the perfect opportunity to get your workout in never presented itself.

The same goes for using these methods to transform your life and attract everything you desire.

Excuses will come whether you want them to or not. And your only hope of winning the battle against them ...is simply expecting them to be there so that when they come, you aren't tricked into rationalizing why you should put any of the techniques off.

Pre-plan ways to do these methods in advance if you have to. For example, if you take public transportation, make sure you've got a pen and pad with you for scripting or gratitude stacking during the ride. And if you drive to work and need both hands on the wheel, hit the record button on your phone and do some spoken scripting instead. And if you're never alone in the car, take a five minute walk by yourself and do it before you leave for the day. Whatever it takes!

Bottomline, this will only work if you stay consistent. And even just five minutes a day of ANY of the methods in this book will do more for you than you could ever imagine. So don't let excuses get in your way. Stay on track.

Strategy 2: Don't Be Overly Critical of Yourself When You First Begin This Process

These techniques are some of the most powerful in the world. And they're extremely easy to do. But holding yourself up to some impossible standard of being perfect with them is a very bad idea.

And it's also another trick your ego likes to play on you.

So don't be hard on yourself if you're ever tempted to slow down. Don't judge yourself if you want to speed up. Until you give yourself a chance to really enjoy doing these every day (and actually start looking forward to them), things like doubt, uncertainty, and impatience might still find a way to intrude on your fun in the very beginning. If this happens and you feel yourself start to waver, don't be overly critical of yourself.

This is the exact time when you should encourage and support yourself instead. Being judgmental of yourself (for any reason) will only slow your progress. But kindness to yourself will speed it up. So don't hold yourself up to some impossible standard. Don't make yourself feel bad if you're not "perfect" with all of this right away. Don't succumb to discouragement. Don't abandon the methods. Don't assume you're not worthy. Don't believe you're not ready. Don't assume the Universe is "against" you. And don't give up on yourself. You're SO much closer to everything you want in life than you could ever realize.

Remember these techniques DO work, they ARE powerful, and they WILL get you where you want to go. Be nice to yourself while you're getting there. It'll make the journey much more enjoyable.

Strategy 3: Prepare for a Rollercoaster of Experiences

Make no mistake - this is going to be FUN. You're going to enjoy the ride. But it's most likely not going to be exactly how you imagined it in your head. And because of this, you need to make sure to stay on course anyway, even when things don't seem to go according to plan.

You want to expect the unexpected here.

In fact, don't be surprised when either your journey OR your results sometimes feel...ordinary. The amazing thing about a lot of this ...is sometimes it doesn't feel amazing.

Even when you manifest something you've waited 20 years for, it's possible it may just feel like another day in your life, while something else that you weren't even worried about might feel absolutely electric when it manifests. You just never know.

Some days might feel very dramatic, while others won't. This is just the ebb and flow of life. Part of the reason for this is that you're going to get better and better at doing all the methods without even realizing how skilled you've become.

Because of this, you'll be much more capable of feeling deeper emotions, but you'll also attract things into your reality so much more effortlessly -- so it won't feel like such a big deal.

So let it be okay for things to feel 'normal' whenever they do. It might happen more than you expect.

But this also doesn't mean you shouldn't expect to feel good every time you do the techniques. They're designed to be fun.

It's just that your good feelings will eventually become your new default mood, and you might get so used to it, that moments of bliss become just another ordinary part of your day (when this happens, you'll be a manifesting machine, and you'll be living an extremely happy life).

It's important to make you aware of this because you'll actually end up feeling better and better and better over time as you continue to experiment with the methods -- but it'll sometimes be a very subtle build-up.

You'll feel great, but it won't be a dramatic increase from how you already felt the day before, so there will be times when it's easy to assume that nothing is happening. But it is happening. Everything is happening.

The main thing to keep in mind is that no matter how 'ordinary' OR 'extraordinary' it feels each day, it's all still working. So just enjoy the rollercoaster while you're on it.

Strategy 4: Keep it Simple - Don't Overthink or Overcomplicate Any of This

Remember, there's always an excuse waiting just around the corner. If this book gave you only one technique, it'd be too easy to rationalize that it wasn't the "best one" and that there just had to be a "better option out there" for you to keep looking for. So I gave you a wider selection of options instead -- each one powerful enough on its own to help you create the vibrational setpoint for anything you want.

But your ego can just as easily slip in and talk you into thinking you have TOO many options and that you never know which one to do. Or you might rationalize that if you spend too much time on one method, you might be sacrificing valuable time you could be spending on another.

The level of mental gymnastics that your ego is capable of is truly miraculous. So this is the perfect time to remind you that once you manifest the life you've been wanting, your ego will fight just as hard to help you keep it (it really IS in your corner!). But until you settle in to a higher and more attractive vibrational frequency, you have to keep things simple at all costs. Remember, this book isn't giving you some giant jigsaw puzzle where you HAVE to use every piece in order to put it all together.

Instead, this book is giving you a menu. So choose whatever item(s) you want from it, whether it's a lot of things, or even only one. Any strategy or method on its own will be more than enough. You get to try them all to see which ones you'd prefer to do more often, but in the end, it doesn't matter which ones you stick with as long as you stick with at least one.

So embrace the truth right now that it doesn't matter which method you choose, how much time you spend on it, or whether it's done "perfectly" or not.

And if you can't decide which technique to use, write them down on little pieces of paper, throw them all in a hat, and pick one. Or flip a coin between your two favorite ones. Whatever you need to do. Just make sure to do something every single day.

That's all you need. Keep it that simple, and everything else will take care of itself.

Strategy 5: Never Make Any of This a Chore

The key to this entire process is that it must never be a chore or inconvenience in any way for you. Ever. Remember, it's not something you "have" to do. It's something you "get" to do.

After all, do you "have" to sit in the first row watching your favorite band perform ...or do you "get" to? Do you "have" to attend the Superbowl or do you "get" to? Is it an obligation or is it a privilege? Is it something you dread or is it something you look forward to?

You've got to be able to make this distinction and do whatever you need to in order to have fun with this. You can think of it as a game, an adventure, an experiment, or anything else if that helps you enjoy the process. Whatever it takes for you to experience it as easy, convenient, engaging, and interesting.

You're growing a muscle here as you play and experiment with this. The methods are already engaging if you give them even half a chance, so just dive in.

The more you do it, the better you get at it -- and the more capacity you have for enjoying it more and more as your life begins to unfold in ways you never could have imagined.

The truth is that you're in this game of life whether you like it or not. And the Law of Attraction is happening right now even if you're not consciously aware of it. So if you're already in the game anyway, you might as well dive in with genuine enthusiasm, take advantage of how the Universe works, make it as fun as you possibly can, and enjoy the ride as you manifest the kind of life you've always wanted!

After all, if the daily journey you go on with these methods isn't fun, you'll never get where you want to go anyway.

Strategy 6: Stop Keeping Score of Where You Are, and Start Focusing on Feeling Good Instead

You have high standards and high expectations of yourself. And nothing you do will ever change this. So it's obviously always going to be tempting to take score of where you are and try to push yourself way further in as short a time as possible. But you're never going to be able to help yourself if you keep looking at where you "are" in relation to your goal and let frustration or disappointment get the better of you if you're not moving as fast as you'd like. In fact, losing patience only reinforces the illusion of being stuck where you are, which then instructs the Universe to keep you there.

You'll actually move WAY faster once you stop trying to force yourself to. And the best way to do that is to move your focus to how you're feeling. The better you feel, the closer your frequency is to what you want to attract. The worse you feel, the further you are. This frightens a lot of people because they suddenly start worrying that any time they feel bad in any way, they're destroying all the progress they've made so far. But it doesn't work like that.

The truth is, positive thoughts are WAY more powerful than negative ones, so you've already got a built-in advantage. And nobody's ever going to feel good ALL the time anyway. And that's okay since this isn't about living up to that impossible standard. It's more about leveraging moments and opportunities for feeling good whenever you can. And since the methods in this book accomplish this for you already, all you have to do is use them on a daily basis, and you're accomplishing everything you need to.

This means that if you try scripting for the first time and you feel like you're being a bit too slow or sluggish, you have to remind yourself that you're not stuck -- you just need a few days of getting used to it.

It's like working out. Nobody bench-presses 300 lbs the first time they go to the gym. But the weight that they DO lift starts triggering positive effects in their body IMMEDIATELY. They may not see the results right away, but progress IS happening.

Along those same lines, you may have only a little fun as you try these methods for the first time, or you might have A LOT right away. Either way, no matter what level of fun you end up experiencing -- focus on it, enjoy it, embrace it, and know that it's making all the difference that you need it to. And stop taking score. You're already way ahead of where you think you are. You'll see.

Strategy 7: Stop Worrying About the Mechanics of Everything Behind the Scenes

So far you've read plenty of explanations in this book of how and why all of this works the way it does. But that's only because most people need some sort of explanation before they give themselves permission to use these methods to manifest their desires. Very few people can just take at face value that IT WORKS.

In the end, though, the only thing that matters is that the manifestation methods do exactly what they're designed for, are simple to understand, and are easy to use. Which means you can put everything else aside and get everything you want if you just simply USE THEM.

The ONLY real value that any of the other information in this book has is if it helps you make that choice to move forward with these powerful techniques.

So don't worry about how it works exactly. Just know that it does. And get to work on it now so that it can start working for you.

Strategy 8: Be as Happy as You Can in the Meantime (It Will Speed Things Up)

Life is beautiful. You don't want to miss out on it just because it's not perfect yet. No matter what's going on in your life at the moment, there are so many things and experiences that you can enjoy RIGHT NOW. So enjoy them.

It's tempting to be impatient with this, especially in the beginning before you realize how much fun you're going to have with the techniques each day. But while you're getting busy manifesting your ideal life, it's important to make sure to take opportunities to enjoy the world around you in the meantime. You're meant to enjoy life NOW, not in some distant future when everything is finally "perfect."

Stop saying to yourself, "I'll be happy when..."

If you wait to be happy, you'll always be waiting.

You need to choose to be happy NOW in any way that you can each and every day. The more you enjoy your life, the faster things will improve anyway. So go to that baseball game. Take that walk in nature. Have that dinner with your friend. Take that dance class. Attend that concert. Have that extra slice of cake. Binge watch that tv show. Treat yourself to that movie.

When you seize these opportunities to live and enjoy your life, you'll naturally end up enjoying the techniques even more every time you use them ...which will then boost your mood and make all these other little moments more enjoyable as well. And your momentum, excitement, and capacity for happiness will all continue to grow as you consistently send the signal to the

Universe that you're happy and that it needs to send you more reasons to keep being happy.

So stop waiting, and be happy now.

Strategy 9: Remember You Have Nothing to Lose and Everything to Gain

There's no risk here in doing any of this. There's no danger. There are no threats.

Doing these exercises every day does absolutely no harm to you whatsoever ...but sticking with them can change your life in ways you never could have dreamed of.

So always remember -- you've got **nothing to lose and everything to gain** by just giving it a try and sticking with it for the next 30 days.

Imagine what you could have accomplished in the last five years if you just took a month out at any point in that period of time to focus your energy and enthusiasm on this. It's worth it.

So do yourself the kindness of finally stepping up and using these manifestation methods to improve every part of your life. You've waited long enough.

Strategy 10: Leave the "How" to the Universe

One of the biggest obstacles to manifestation is thinking "How will this happen?"

But you don't need to know. Your job is to have the desire, set the intention, keep your vibration up (using the manifestation methods you've learned), and be open to signs and opportunities from the Universe along the way.

The how, the where, the why, and the when are NOT your job. That will all come to you.

YOUR POWER IS IN THE 'NOW'
-- NOT IN THE 'HOW'

The Universe is ALWAYS looking out for you, even when you don't see it. But you've got to leave it room to do the work, and you must trust it to handle whatever you're unable to do.

Knowing when to take your hand off the wheel and let the Universe do the heavy lifting is one of the biggest differences between people who successfully attract the things that they want ...and people who bang their heads against the wall, day after day, wondering why nothing is happening for them.

After all, you can leave a message for a company you want to work for, but you can't force them to call you back. You can practice a performance AND deliver it to perfection, but you can't make the audience cheer. And you can take an umbrella to the park, but you can't make it rain.

And even when certain things seem like they're in your control, that doesn't always mean you have to (or even should) do any of the work.

After all, for every 1 or 2 ways of succeeding that you see in front of you, the Universe has at least 100 better ones just waiting around the corner.

And the Universe always knows what your path of least resistance is to attracting whatever you want.

The possibilities for all the good that can come into your life really are endless. They always have been.

And oftentimes, whatever you think you want, the Universe might have something even better in store for you that you actually would have wished for -- if only you believed something that great was really possible.

So relax and let the Universe take care of the 'How'. Let it handle the timing of everything and trust that whatever you need WILL come.

As for knowing whether you should sit in an empty room meditating on what you want ...or whether you should physically do something instead, it all depends on what's in your control and whether it feels good or not. You're going to take action in at least some ways, of course. You're on a physical plane of existence after all. The key distinction is that you're going to want to take action from a mindset of abundance, not one of scarcity.

If you're trying to 'force' something with your action, you're actually fighting against yourself and screaming to the Universe that you don't have what you want yet (which only invites more of the same). But when you're acting from a mindset of abundance, you're telling the Universe that everything is okay, which frees it up to give you what you want.

Ultimately, your only job ...is to focus your attention on what you desire, let the energies that match it line up ...and take action when it makes sense, when it's in your sphere of control, and when it seems easy and fun to do. Struggling or trying to 'force' things to happen will only slow them down.

The purpose behind the techniques in this book comes down to one thing: making sure you're focusing on what you want MORE THAN focusing on what you don't want (or the lack of what you want). So just let go of trying to make it happen, use the techniques to relax and let it happen, and sit back and relax as everything begins working out for you.

And just in case you still need a little more motivation to keep up with all of this, the following chapter will walk you through an easy mental exercise for helping you discover your big "WHY" so you can stick with it and finally manifest the life you've always wanted.

Chapter 28: Finding A "Why" That Makes Everything Work

When something you want feels impossible to achieve, it's unfortunately way too easy to get discouraged and quit before you even give yourself a chance to get it.

This is why so many people fail to attract what they want, even after they've learned exactly how to do it. They let themselves believe that everything they want the most will always be just out of reach no matter what they do.

If they only realized how close they were to getting what they wanted this entire time.

The truth is the Universe desperately WANTS you to have your every last wish. It's practically begging you to step up just a LITTLE and meet it halfway. If you look for signs of this, they're all around you.

Why do you think these techniques are so simple?

Why would it possibly be this easy?

Because it was always meant to be.

The Universe is motivated by expansion. It loves speed. It loves possibility. When anyone wants anything, the Universe automatically expands in response. The bigger the desire, the more the Universe gets to "be". This is why it wants to do everything it can to give you your desires. You've already helped the Universe expand with all the things you're currently wishing for.

But only when you actually achieve those first initial goals will you allow yourself to dream even bigger dreams and trigger the Universe to expand even more as it vibrationally constructs all those new possibilities.

That's why the Universe does so much of the heavy lifting for you. All the moments of inspiration, coincidences, chance meetings, brilliant ideas that pop into your head, and other positive circumstances are freely given to you as a gift to help you manifest your goals and inspire you to create even more possibilities with even bigger dreams.

But despite everything it can do, the Universe is still governed by the Law of Attraction. And since you still have free will, the ONE thing the Universe can't do is make your choices for you. No matter how easy and fun the methods are, the Universe can't make you "want" your desires enough to do them every day.

This means that the question of whether you succeed or fail still comes down to basic human psychology. You need to take advantage of the way your mind works and make these techniques a fun, enjoyable, and inevitable part of your day.

In other words, you need to find a way to motivate yourself enough to do them consistently.

It's like working out. If you're not inspired enough to do it regularly, you're just not going to see any results. This is where your big "WHY" comes in.

Your big "why" is actually HOW all of this is going to finally come together for you.

You need a reason that leaves no room for silly excuses, no concern over how long it might take, and no chance that you're going to ignore what's possible for your life this time. You found your way to this book because you knew that the Law of Attraction works, and all you needed was a way to make it work FOR YOU. Now that it's clear you've finally found it, think back on all you could have accomplished in the past year if you had been consistently doing these techniques with genuine enthusiasm the entire time. Really think about this.

Now think back to all you could have done in the past three years. The past five.

Now think how much better it could have been if you started ten years ago. Think about all the improvements in your health, your finances, your relationships, your career. Even just your day-to-day moment-to-moment happiness. Think about it.

Think of all the miracles that would have unfolded by now. How much different and better could everything already be for you? What could already be yours? And what if it all could STILL be yours ...RIGHT NOW -- if only you finally just STARTED? Started using the methods. Started allowing yourself to enjoy them and really dive in. Started committing to having the life you've always desired.

How much higher would your salary be?

How much bigger would your business be?

Would you be happily married?

Would you be happily remarried?

Would you be living by the beach?

Would you have multiple homes?

Would you be inspiring others every day?

Would you wake up each morning with a true sense of ease, hope, and joy?

Would confidence and satisfaction be your default state of being?

Would happiness, excitement, and enthusiasm be emotions you got to experience all the time?

Now think about how your life is right now ...and look a year into the future of what your life will be if nothing changes.

Fives years. Ten years. Twenty years!

What's it going to cost you if you ignore this opportunity to finally start using these easy and convenient methods the way they were always meant to be used? What's your life going to be like if you throw this gift away and go back to the way you've already been doing things?

What will you be missing out on by leaving your life up to chance ...when you can just as easily take control, be intentional about what you want to attract, and enjoy all the things in life you so richly deserve?

You Know Why You're Here

And You Know Why You Found This Book.

Why did you buy this book (and every book and program before it)? What was the result you were looking for? What was your hope for the future? What was your vision? Why are you reading this right now? Whatever the answer is, THAT is your big 'why'. Write it down. Read it to yourself every morning and every night. Have it memorized for every time you try out one of the techniques. It's your reason to keep going.

And it's valid. No matter what it is. It's the most valid thing in the world. YOU are the most valid person in the world. No matter what anyone has ever told you in the past (including yourself), you deserve to have everything you've ever wanted.

But you have to claim it. And the only way to claim it is by doing the manifestation methods you now have in your possession.

They're already easy to use.

They already work.

And the Universe is already prepared to handle everything else for you (and I mean EVERYthing).

The only thing you have to do ...is choose to finally have everything you've ever wanted.

Look to your 'Why' every day. And choose.

IT'S THAT SIMPLE.

And now that you have your big 'Why' to push forward with, it's time to finally settle the question once and for all of whether you're truly worthy of having the life you've always dreamt of...

Chapter 29: Making Yourself Worthy (And Making Sure the Universe Knows It)

As I was writing the first draft of this book, I went through a lot of different ideas for how I wanted to title this chapter, even though the content itself was always going to be the same.

Just a couple of examples (of at least ten ideas I was choosing from) include:

"Are you worthy of having everything you want?"

"How to tell if you're worthy or not."

"You're already worthy! Here's why."

So why did I finally settle on "Making Yourself Worthy" (And Making Sure The Universe Knows It)?"

Because 99% of people who learn about the Law of Attraction always seem to be under some false impression that they have to "do" something in order to deserve happiness and success. This is all in spite of being told by almost every book or program out there that they're ALREADY worthy. They refuse to accept that they don't still have something to prove. They don't recognize that just by being born, they've already paid every last one of their dues for receiving the life of their dreams.

This is human nature, of course. Getting "something for nothing" doesn't really compute for us because our standards for survival on this physical plane always involve some form of exchange.

In other words, we assume that if we want to "get" ...then we need to "give" in return.

The issue here is that we already ARE giving. We just don't realize it. We don't see it because the "giving" that's required isn't in the form that we're used to. Our "giving" is being accomplished by having desires that automatically provide the Universe with the opportunity to expand in response to them. In other words, our work is already done.

But even if we understand this on an intellectual level, we've still got the ego creeping in the background doubting the truth of this anyway. And that's why you never seem to get very far with any of this.

That nagging suspicion that "it can't be this easy!" or "there's no way it's so simple!" is EXACTLY the reason that it hasn't been "easy" or "simple" for you yet.

If you could only just know in your heart of hearts how much the Universe loves you, how much it really is in your corner, how much it wants you to have what you want, and how quickly this can all really happen for you -- your head would spin, and you'd barge in on every person you love, shove a copy of this book in their face, and tell them to just try the methods out already.

Here's the thing -- since there's most likely a very important and influential part of your mind that refuses to accept that you're already worthy -- then we need to find a way for you to "earn" it in terms that you can accept. But these terms ALSO need to add to the quality of your life (so that you're in the proper frequency to receive your desires).

You're already worthy. And the Universe knows it. Now it's time for you to finally know it as well. At your deepest level of being. To really 'get' that there's no shortage of good. There's only abundance. You need to readjust your perspective so that feeling selfish becomes impossible and feeling worthy is inevitable. And it's easier to do than you think.

Here are 2 highly-effective ways of achieving this improved state of being:

#1 - Live A Mission in Service to More Than Just Yourself

This doesn't mean that you need to commit to some ambitious cause that will demand all of your time, energy, and money. You don't have to move to a new city. You don't have to change your lifestyle. You don't even have to volunteer for anything.

You simply need to remember that we're surrounded by more than what our senses detect. We're literally swimming in energy. And we can effect that energy through our intentions, our moods, and our emotions.

So make the choice to live your every moment as a source of positivity to all of those around you -- whether you know them or not, and whether you physically interact with them or not.

Be willing to serve as a vehicle of light for anyone who might need it, no matter what form that might take. It can be through action OR through stillness.

You get to decide.

But however it might appear in any given moment, you are essentially committing to being a conduit for love, light, positivity, possibility, abundance, warmth, compassion, support, strength, and joy.

When you walk into a room, you literally radiate the energy of any or all of those qualities. That is the impact you make on everyone and everything around you. You make your world a better place through this intention. You brighten the mood of others without them even realizing it was you. You intend happiness and success for all of those around you.

When walking in nature and passing trees gently swaying in the breeze, you acknowledge them and understand that their swaying is just the Universe saying "hi, I love you."

Silently return the sentiment with your thoughts. Commit to being the kind of person who supports others when they need it. Be the kind of person who says something kind to a stranger when it's clear they're having a bad day and could use a quick pick-me-up.

Live your life with a code of honor that you consider fair and just, even if others are unable to live up to the same standard. Begin each day with this intention. Literally say out loud "I commit to being a vehicle of love today. I am here to radiate positivity and joy, and to offer those around me good feelings, hope, faith, relief, confidence, and any other energetic support they might need. I know I will come into contact with the perfect people who can contribute to my well-being just as much as I can contribute to theirs. And if I don't see how they can help me, it doesn't matter. I'm a wonderful person who brings ease and joy wherever they go, and I leave the rest up to the Universe"

Feel free to take real action as well. Do good things -- but only choose things that truly make you feel good.

If volunteering for ten hours in a soup kitchen feels like a chore, then don't do it. Everything you do should always feel good because that's the frequency that invites everything you want to manifest.

And there are plenty of other ways of doing good for others that you can enjoy while still making a difference.

It's all about feeling good as you do this. Of course, you're most likely not going to feel good 100% of the time, and that's okay -- especially since positive emotions are always more powerful than negative ones, so you can easily tip the scales of receiving in your favor. But just because good outweighs bad, that doesn't mean you should voluntarily allow bad experiences when you can just as easily have good ones instead.

So you need to do nice things for others that also feel good to you. You're not being selfish or petty or unfair by requiring that you enjoy it. If anything, you're being selfLESS because when you enjoy doing something nice for someone else, you're going to want to do it even more, so you end up helping more people more of the time. The Universe loves win-win situations, so give it what it wants.

For example, if you've got a few bucks to spare per week, you can take a sticky notepad, write a quick hopeful message, stick the note to a dollar bill, and hide it on a supermarket shelf each day, where a stranger will stumble on it.

Imagine the relief and joy you'll give someone who's having a bad day when they find the dollar and a note that reads:

"This is your reminder that you are loved, money and success are just around the corner waiting for you, and you deserve every last bit of it."

...or "This is your reminder that you are loved."

...or "Miracles happen."

...or "You found this note because you're awesome."

...or "You were meant to find this. You're also meant for more happiness and success than you could ever imagine."

Or anything else that inspires hope, faith, or simply a smile.

You can use this 'good deed' as a manifestation method as well. As you put that dollar with the note in the supermarket shelf, view it as an investment with compounding universal interest -- and visualize/intend it multiplying by tens or even hundreds, and finding its way back to you (in some pleasant way that the Universe will decide).

Based on this one example alone, it's obvious that it's easy to do at least one kind thing for someone else every day, even if you don't know them.

It could be as simple as sharing a recipe, giving a kind word, recommending a book you love to someone who really needs it, buying a book for someone because you know they'll never do it on their own, or showing kindness in any other way.

Regardless of how much or how little real action you take, make it your mission to make the Universe a better place just by being here. See yourself as a vehicle to inspire others, to bring abundance, to be a beacon of light that anyone can sense in their own unique way.

You're a spiritual warrior fighting for the happiness and ease of all those around you. But you don't need any weapon because you are the weapon. You are the sword that cuts through negativity with just your intention. You show people with your presence alone --without having to say a single word -- that life is a miracle ...and so are they.

The self-worth you experience through this process is so healthy that it makes it literally impossible to judge yourself or feel bad about who you are in any way.

You automatically become a better version of yourself. You experience a renewed confidence. You finally recognize a sense of worthiness you never thought you could ever access. And the frequency you vibrate at when this happens is so magnetic, the floodgates begin to fly open because the Universe recognizes how genuine you're being as you do this for others.

And just feeling good from all of this will help you effortlessly radiate a frequency of joy, which will then elevate everyone around you.

Know this -- a healthy and powerful you is the best thing that could ever happen to anyone else because from that position of positive influence, you're much more capable of helping them when they really need it.

So manifesting what you want actually makes the world a better place. And by realizing this, you attract it faster, you enjoy it more deeply, you discover more resources, and you help both yourself and others way more than you ever could have hoped. The best part is -- you're also blazing the trail and making it easier for others to follow in your footsteps and manifest everything they want in life as well.

This is also why you always remember to extend this very same level of kindness ...to yourself. There's nobody in the world more suited to helping you ...than yourself. This brings us to the next highly-effective way of pushing self-judgment to the side and inviting self-worth instead.

#2 - Be Open to The Possibility That Things Have Always Been Better Than They Seemed

As human beings, we tend to think we know everything. Again, it's a survival mechanism. If we can make a clear and final decision on something (especially something important), we can file that in our minds in a predictable way to base all of our other choices off of.

If you see a poisonous cobra in front of a plate of potato chips, you don't have to expend very much mental energy processing whether it's worth the risk to go near them. And if you see an adorable little kitten there instead, your decision is the opposite, but just as easy. But again, we don't always know the 'right' answer. 500 years ago, we thought the earth was flat. 100 years ago, we thought air travel was impossible for anything except birds. And today, we still believe we have to struggle and suffer in order to get what we want.

But is that really true? Genuinely ask yourself this question and be open to the possibility that it's not what you've been raised to believe.

If you were told growing up that airplanes were an impossible concept, would that stop them from still existing right now? Of course not. And you'd be in for quite a shock when someone finally told you about them.

So maybe it's time to consider the possibility (or, let's be honest -- the truth) that you really are worthy, you always were worthy, this is really how the Universe works, and until now, you simply weren't aware of it.

Maybe it's time to admit that we unreasonably hold onto outdated beliefs because our ego is worried about what might happen if we adapt.

Maybe it's time to take a look in the mirror and realize that, while they were only looking out for our best interests -- many authorities in our lives have inadvertently conditioned us to think we're not good enough. Perhaps a passing comment from a school teacher (who was only trying to teach a lesson) could have easily scarred our self-esteem when we were way too young to recognize it was happening.

And if that's what really happened, maybe it's time to stop allowing that moment to dictate your entire life.

You are pure light. Positive vibrant energy.

An individualization of god.

You're worthy simply by the fact that you exist.

Your desire is literally god speaking through you.

If you only knew how important you really are and what you mean to the Universe, you'd be astonished. So embrace your worthiness. Give yourself the gift of trying these methods. Do this for yourself. Do it for your loved ones. Do it for the world around you. Do it for the Universe.

You're serving ALL interests through this choice, and you're being rewarded for it in a way that ANYONE can enjoy, but few actually allow themselves to. You're already worthy.

And as you're about to read in the next chapter ahead, you were chosen to live a brilliant life a long time ago.

Chapter 30: You've Been Chosen

You've waited long enough. The Universe chose you to be happy, successful, and fulfilled a long time ago. And now it's time.

IT'S TIME TO FINALLY

HAVE WHAT YOU WANT

It's time to be who you've always wanted to be, have what you've always wanted to have, and do what you've always wanted to do.

It's time to enjoy the rewards you earned a long time ago through your patience, your effort, and your undeniable resilience all these years.

It's time for friendships that enrich your life, experiences that take your breath away, and moments of genuine joy and fulfillment.

It's time to love and be loved on profound levels that could never be described, to overcome every last challenge with complete and total ease, and to play the game of life at a level never thought possible. It's time to breathe easy knowing your days of worry and stress over finances, relationships, and health can finally now end.

It's time to start treating yourself with the care, kindness, and respect you've always deserved. To take every opportunity to stop and smell the roses, dance in the rain, pet that friendly dog, take that awesome vacation, play on that beautiful beach, go on that perfect picnic, buy that dream home, hug that special someone, and just LIVE.

It's time. And this book is the blueprint for sculpting that reality and creating your magnificent life.

The best part is that the manifestation methods you've learned can easily work in any combination you put them in OR can be enough all on their own. If you only liked one of them and stuck with it, that would be everything you ever needed. But first you have to use it.

IT'S TIME TO FINALLY START
USING WHAT YOU'VE LEARNED

The time for research and theory is over. And the time for putting everything you've learned into practice has officially arrived.

The methods in this book WORK. But you have to decide that you want this enough to actually use them. You have to choose.

Nobody can do this for you. It has to be you.

And by choosing to practice any or all of these techniques, you're sending a powerful, definite, unequivocal, undeniable, and unapologetic message to yourself AND to the Universe that you're READY.

The key to remember here is that any little thing that you do just once a day is going to make a difference. And the momentum you'll pick up once it starts working will amaze you. As long as you stay with it, this momentum will never stop. It'll just keep getting better and better with every passing day.

But you have to begin.

Drop everything else that isn't essential to your life. Drop every distraction. Drop everything extra that's overwhelming you. Disregard all the conflicts, all the headaches, and all the complications. Put every other book and program on the shelf and use what's right in front of you. It's more than enough to get you where you want to be.

Finally, don't allow any of your perceived limitations to keep you from doing this.

IT'S TIME TO PUT YOUR LIMITATIONS ON HOLD

You can do this if only you give yourself the chance. So put all your old ideas about how things are "supposed to be" on hold, and suspend your disbelief for the next 30 days to just see what happens. Any nudges of doubt, feelings of hopelessness, and notions that none of this is really possible are only just distractions that your ego is throwing in front of you because it's afraid. Any limitations you see are nothing more than persistent illusions that are no longer serving you. They're clusters of energy transformed in a specific way to match perceptions you've been holding onto.

If the Universe can create the planets and the stars and EVERYTHING around you, it can EASILY create anything else you want in it, too. It can create the money. It can create the relationship. It can create the health. It can create the success. It can create it all.

This isn't actually overwhelming. This isn't actually complicated. This isn't too big for you to handle. This isn't out of your reach. Don't be fooled by any notion that tells you otherwise.

The Universe really is a friendly place. Everything you want is yours to have.

THIS WORKS IF YOU WORK IT!

Don't let the negativity of other people stop you from moving forward with this. If there are people in your life who might scoff at any of these ideas, don't tell them what you're doing. Just move forward with it.

Before long, they'll see the results as clearly as you do, and they'll be asking you what your secret is.

Above all else, remember -- you can do this! You ARE doing this. You're creating your entire life already, whether you like it or not. So you might as well be intentional about it. You might as well acknowledge the truth that you are a divine being connected to everything and everyone around you -- with access to every single bit of energy that exists in the Universe.

You might as well embrace the truth that great things are meant to unfold in your life.

And because you are already so POWERFUL (and always have been), the ONLY thing that stops you from having what you want is your false belief that you're only what you see in the mirror, that you don't deserve more, and that it can't be yours.

Break the false pattern by using the methods in this book to take conscious control of what you're letting yourself think about. Let them help you consciously create habits that will produce the amazing life you want to live.

Remember, most people aren't living the life they want. They're only living what they think they're capable of, what they think they're worthy of, and what they think they're allowed to have by some phony mysterious invisible force that's holding them back and keeping them from their happiness. Don't fall for such a destructive illusion.

You're in an abundant Universe that's here to support you with every single breath you take. Affirm to yourself "I am always attracting more abundance, more joy, and even more wealth!"

Once you do that, the floodgates will open and you'll wonder in amazement where all of these wonderful experiences were this entire time.

And you'll continue to manifest your dream life with each and every new day from now on. But nothing happens without your choice to move forward and do this.

IT'S TIME TO CHOOSE

Every single circumstance of your life can change however you want it to. Your entire life is in your hands. You're more than you ever realized. You are infinite. Reclaim your power. Declare to the Universe that you've chosen a new and better reality ...and it will be yours.

Know what you want and simply go after it. Don't ask anyone's permission. Just use the gratitude, scripting, and visualization methods in this book to shift your energy, adjust your signal, and attract whatever you want. The time is now and the moment is yours. GO FOR IT.

All things are possible, so stop playing small.

You can literally help awaken human consciousness and make the world a better place by simply living from your true nature and manifesting the most magnificent life possible. Stay on the path. For you and everyone around you.

You owe this to yourself.

Everything you need is already here. And it's simpler and easier than you ever could have imagined.

Whatever you think about and focus on the most WILL materialize. And the techniques in this book are specifically designed to help you put your attention on what you want in a way that will energize, excite, and thrill you.

You'll easily use them to think more about what you DO want and less about what you DON'T. And at the end of the day, that's the ONLY thing you ever really have to worry about.

If all you ever did was think about the things you're grateful for, you'd succeed in every important part of your life. If all you did was script what you wanted through the written or spoken word, it would all come to you.

And if all you did was visualize the outcome with gratitude while disregarding the "how" behind it, nothing could stop it from getting to you. Opportunities would emerge, events would unfold, and circumstances would shift in wonderful ways as you line up with the energy of what you want and pull it into your reality.

Remember, gratitude for anything at any moment tells the Universe that good things happen to you, which automatically instructs the Universe to send you more of the same!

But in order for this to finally happen for you, you must acknowledge the core truth that this DOES work, you ARE worthy, and you CAN do it! And any idea in conflict with that is just a lie that somehow found its way to you a long time ago.

IT'S TIME TO LIVE THE LIFE
YOU'VE ALWAYS WANTED

There's always going to be an excuse to not be happy.

But you can't expect anything to ever really change if you keep buying into those excuses and continue to rationalize to yourself the idea of "I'll be happy when..."

You'll only delay that happiness forever.

Don't let this be another Law of Attraction book that you throw on the shelf after trying it out for only a few days. Break that cycle now. **You found this book for a reason.**

No matter how many mistakes you make, no matter what you think of yourself, the Universe loves you.

It will move heaven and earth to give you anything and everything you want at the drop of a hat. It will move through every moment, every person, and every circumstance it needs to in order to fulfill your every wish.

All it needs from you is to send it the right instructions.

All it needs is for you to place your order.

Use any or all of the manifestation methods in this book to finally do this for yourself and make having everything you want your default point of attraction once and for all. And then confidently go about each day resting in the certainty that what you want is yours.

And sit back and watch as it joyfully erupts into your reality.

You're a powerful, potent, magnificent magnetic being.

Great things are going to happen for you today.

Relax. Trust. Let it in. It'll happen, friend. It's already happening. And the faster you let go, the quicker it'll come.

You have the power to change ANYTHING.

You were chosen for this.

It's time.

Epilogue: Gravity of the Cosmos

Now that you realize how important it is for you to make this happen in your life …and now that you understand the kind of miraculous experiences you can enjoy if you just begin in a healthy smart way …there's only one question left:

"What now?"

Naturally, you're ready to dive in and start making this happen, but you're still not sure about what you should do next. In this final portion of the book, I want to answer this question for you and help you kick things off on the right foot by giving you some high-impact extra bonuses that are designed to help you get started on this right away.

The first bonus is a short document I created, titled **"The First 10 Days."** I've kept it very basic so there's no guesswork needed, but it's basically a 10-day calendar of suggested methods you can do each day in an order that's comfortable, simple, and easy.

And just so you don't feel stuck on only one option (since you're obviously looking for a sequence that works well for you personally), I'm giving you four different combinations of this calendar.

One (or more) of them will surely work as a starting point for you, regardless of your individual preferences. After all, some people like to do a lot of scripting right away. Others prefer to stick mostly with gratitude exercises. And some even like to have at least one or two days of using the Walking Meditation technique.

Whatever is best suited for you, you'll have it as an option.

But I don't want to just leave you with that one bonus alone. I'm also giving you **"The Elite Five"**-- my own personal list of favorite manifestation methods to use.

All of the methods in this book are wonderful. And they all work. But I'm often asked which ones I enjoy doing the most myself, so in case any new readers are curious about this as well, I've decided to share it with you. The list may surprise you.

All you need to do to get these 2 bonuses is go to **www.LastLOABook.com** and claim them there.

But before you do that, I also want to get you access to a very special live training that I occasionally give to readers.

It's called: **"3 Secrets For Manifesting Your Desires *Faster Than You Ever Thought Possible* ...Without Losing Patience, Losing Hope, or Losing Your Way."**

Any time someone comes to me searching for a clear way to finally turn things around and begin attracting the things that are most important to them -- no matter how many times they may have failed in the past -- the content in this training is always the information that I share with them.

The details that I provide are my absolute best advice for manifesting your deepest desires and creating a life that you truly love.

I go very deep on this presentation, but I still manage to keep it extremely straightforward so that anyone who's already familiar with everything I've covered in this book will be able to easily understand it and use everything I teach.

I even share important details from my own story of how I used the Law of Attraction to turn things around when everything in my own life was going in the worst possible direction. You'll learn a little more about how I know what I know, why I know it, and how I've used this information to prove to myself that this always works with flawless precision.

These details weren't necessary for the book, so I didn't want to make it longer than it needed to be, but they really hammer home some crucial points in the training, and I'm confident that the things I share about myself will be very useful to you.

You'll understand what I mean once you get a chance to watch it. I can't recommend it highly enough, which is why I wanted to make sure you had a chance to view it.

Just as with the other bonuses, all you have to do to access this training is go to www.LastLOABook.com and follow the easy instructions for getting your hands on it free of charge.

Finally, before we get to the last huge bonus I've prepared for you …I want to quickly talk about the title for this chapter: "Gravity of the Cosmos."

What does that even mean?

Well, when you do a little research, you'll discover that the word 'cosmos' is often interchangeable with the word 'universe' -- but with one clear difference:

Using the word cosmos implies a universe that has a very specific "order" to it.

It's a universe without chaos -- an orderly system or entity that's governed by a clear level of predictability …IF you understand it.

There's still a lot of complexity, of course, but there's also clarity and purpose. It's something you can figure out. It's something you can calculate. There's a cause and effect quality to it.

In other words, while you can't completely control it 100%, you CAN heavily influence how you experience it -- as long as you understand how it works.

And the only 'rule' you need to know and understand in order to successfully do this ...is the Law of Attraction.

This brings us to 'gravity.'

Most people think of gravity as little more than a force of nature that keeps them firmly set on the ground. But it's obviously much more than that.

It actually describes an invisible yet natural phenomenon by which ALL things with mass or energy are pulled toward one another. This includes planets, stars, even entire galaxies. It even includes things like sound and light. It's that deep.

And remember, everything is energy, so there's a "gravity" to everything that exists. This is actually where the phrase "like attracts like" comes from. So what we're really talking about here is the process of pulling what you want into your life in a way that's in harmony with the order and balance of the Universe.

And that's why when I was putting together my advanced level 90-day program for manifesting your desires through the Law of Attraction -- I could think of no better title for the project than "Gravity of the Cosmos."

Each part of the program was built on the recognition that there's always a way to understand how the Universe works -- that when properly identified -- allows you to leverage its power to pull desired events, experiences, and people into your physical reality at will.

You manifest money, relationships, health, success -- everything -- by pushing the right buttons in the right order. It's that simple.

After all, now that you've got these wonderfully dynamic techniques at your disposal, you want to be organized and efficient in how you use them.

"Gravity of the Cosmos" helps you do this for up to 90 days so you can comfortably build a daily habit of using the Law of Attraction in an enjoyable way without ever being overwhelmed, losing focus of your goal, or wondering what to do next.

By delivering the content in bite-sized pieces, the program ensures that nothing ever feels too big, no method ever becomes unmanageable, and no lifestyle is ever too complicated to fit this daily routine into.

Everything is kept simple, easy, and seamless.

This is the program that people turn to when they need expert guidance on structuring a daily calendar for the methods in this book. It's where they go when they need the perfect combination of insight, encouragement, assistance, and effectiveness.

And as my gift to you, I'm giving you the first couple days of this groundbreaking program for FREE.

That's right, as a thank you for being a new reader of mine, I'm giving you a free look into this unique project and allowing you to access the first part of it so that you can get that perfect boost of momentum and start using the Law of Attraction in the easiest and most beneficial way -- right now with no further delay.

That way, even if you never get your hands on the entire program, you'll still at least have this solid foundation and early game plan to go 30, 60, or even 90 straight days on your own.

These first couple of days that I give you will serve as their own specialized mini-program. Knowing that the ego hates commitment, I actually built key benchmarks into the entire project.

After all, we both know that 90 days might sound too ambitious for some people on the surface. Even 60 might sound like a lot (until they realize how much fun each day is, of course).

So the program is actually chunked into 30-day sections, and each of those sections are chunked into 10-day segments as well.

That way, users have the opportunity to build momentum in much more manageable timeframes, but by the time they're finished, they still end up getting 90 full days of amazing energetic shifts and consistent increasing progress.

I segmented the first couple of days as well in order to make this bonus for you really special. You'll be able to dive right in today and finally begin enjoying the process of manifesting what you want through the techniques you've learned.

And the best part is you're getting something that's been designed and built off of a lot of genuine feedback and experience. I know what it's like to deal with this personally. And I know what it's like to help others deal with this as well. In fact, when I first started working with people privately, the #1 thing they always requested was a day-to-day guided schedule they could easily follow that WORKS.

So as soon as I knew for sure that the methods you learned in this book were advanced enough to support such an ambitious project, I went straight to work creating it.

But I also added all sorts of extra pieces that I knew would help -- including key insights for sticking with the process, proper encouragement when it was needed, and -- most importantly -- strategic advice for making sure things always made sense as the user went further into the program and started seeing more results.

I realized that some people wouldn't instantly recognize the power or value of all the methods (or that they'd be a little hesitant to try some of them), so I inserted all of them in a user-friendly way throughout the entire experience.

The Mission Accomplished Method.

The Instant Replay Method.

The Protecting the Prize Method.

They're all there -- along with a few other tricks that didn't make it into the book because they made a lot more sense as audio or video presentations, rather than instructions on a printed page.

You'll get to dive more deeply into everything you just learned in this book (and a whole lot more) in a clear, organized, easy way without having to worry about missing anything or wondering what to do next.

By building out the program this way, I knew I could guarantee both variety AND consistency for anyone going through it. It's all about making the process engaging, but it's also about making it simple to follow along with.

I obviously wanted something that's enjoyable, dependable, and easy to do. But more than that, what I really wanted was to design the perfect program for customizing the user's schedule and lifestyle around -- and ensure they could finally make this work, enjoy a healthy and reliable routine, and fully succeed in attracting and manifesting the things that they wanted.

Remember, the whole key is to do these methods consistently.

And the only way that's ever going to happen is if you actually enjoy them, get enough real results to stay encouraged, and have a way to stick with it that never feels like some overwhelming chore.

That's the vision I held to as I created this program.

Unless you work with me personally for 3 months at a rate of at least $25K, this program is the only way to get this level of insight and immersion, and there is absolutely no higher value I'm currently able to offer on this type of scale.

If you're finally ready to dive into these methods to manifest the life you know you deserve, but you're still not sure where to begin for any reason, Gravity of the Cosmos was built for you.

That's why when you dive into these first couple of days that I'm giving you, you'll notice there's nothing fancy or complicated about it. It's been designed to fit into your lifestyle in a comfortable and sensible way.

So please enjoy the first couple of days with my compliments.

Again, you can get your hands on this bonus along with all the others by going to www.LastLOABook.com.

I'm also going to stay in touch and send you a little extra support over email here and there. It might be a powerful bonus technique that didn't fit in with this book's topics. Or it might be a quick note of encouragement or new insight I've discovered. Or it might just be a really cool surprise that I wanted to share that I knew you'd really enjoy.

Either way, I know what it's like to struggle with this, and I know how to win, so the idea of helping others like me get where they want to go fills me with more joy than I could ever describe.

I want only good things for you, and my goal will always be to help you achieve the happiness and success you so richly deserve, and if I can help you with that on your journey, I know I've done my job.

Finally, as I mentioned at the beginning of this book, you're also getting a bonus chapter that I wrote after I had already completed this book, titled **"Knowing When To Hand Over Control And Let The Universe Do The Work For You."**

It's one of my absolute favorite Law of Attraction explanations, and I know you're going to love it.

So to recap, I'm giving you a total of 5 additional resources to help you get started working in harmony with the Law of Attraction the way you were always meant to...

- "The First 10 Days" Daily Schedule of Law of Attraction Techniques

- "The Elite Five" Top Recommended Manifestation Methods

- Advanced Training: "Accessing the Perfect Frequency For Manifesting Your Desires ...Without Losing Patience, Losing Hope, or Losing Your Way."

- "Gravity of the Cosmos" Advanced Level Full Immersion 90-Day Guided Program - Special Insider Preview

- Extra Bonus Chapter: "Knowing When To Hand Over Control And Let The Universe Do The Work For You."

Please enjoy them all. Here's the link one more time where you can get them:

www.LASTLOABOOK.com

Above all else, always remember the Universe is in your corner. Always remember it wants you to have everything you've ever wished for so that you can wish for even more.

It loves possibility.

It loves expansion.

And it loves you.

Watch for those manifestation raindrops.

Enjoy that ice cream.

Glide on that skateboard.

There's so much in the world waiting to be enjoyed by you.

It's JUST out of sync vibrationally as you read this.

But it's still within your reach.

Use the manifestation methods you now have access to. Take advantage of all the bonuses I just gave you. Play the game to win. Enjoy the ride. And remember you are more loved and supported than you'll ever realize.

You came here to create. You came here to thrive. You came here to smile, laugh, love and LIVE.

Start now.

There's no better time.

A QUICK NOTE FROM ANDREW:

Thank you so much for reading.

If you found this book helpful, please review and share it.

That helps it find its way to those who need it.

This would mean a lot to me. Thank You.

www.ingramcontent.com/pod-product-compliance
Lightning Source LLC
Chambersburg PA
CBHW030906080526
44589CB00010B/165